The Sweet Potato Diet was first introduced to me via Snapchat when I saw Michael eating sweet potatoes and chicken in the Morellifit Snapchat. This diet has changed my life because it hasn't just saved me a ton of money, but has given me all I need in order to have a better quality of life as well as a great healthy meal option that I enjoy eating. I've always loved sweet potatoes and didn't know that you could eat them every day and eat them in many different ways, which is good when you're a college student on a budget. Thanks to Michael and his Sweet Potato Diet I have saved a lot of money while eating something that has great nutritional value and helped me achieve my fitness goals.

—JORGE H.

The Sweet Potato Diet changed my life in so many ways. Once I removed all other carb sources from my diet, I was able to jump-start my weight loss when I hit a plateau. I lost 6 pounds in the first week. Sweet potatoes are the only carb I will eat now! I also got my youngest son Jacob eating sweet potatoes. He is a type 1 diabetic and sweet potatoes are a great complex carb and do not spike insulin levels and that helps keep his numbers from dramatic swings!! Sweet potatoes are a gift from God in a neat little package! *The Sweet Potato Diet* is a gift from Morellifit!!

—BILL M.

The Sweet Potato Diet changed my life. I was always eating clean. Protein, veggies, and healthy fats. Maybe a sweet potato here and there. I started incorporating sweet potatoes in every meal, and I saw a change in my body and how I felt. They also left me full and satisfied. I believe sweet potatoes are a hidden gem. Most people don't really know much about them. Sweet potatoes even satisfied my sweet tooth!

—DANIELLE M.

If there was one thing that broke my fat loss plateau, it was Michael's Sweet Potato Diet. When I first started I lost an incredible 7 pounds in 7 days with no exercise, just this change in diet! Moving forward I lost a total of 20 pounds in 45 days and I'm happy to say the Sweet Potato Diet has become everyday life for me!

—NICK G

I was first introduced to the Sweet Potato Diet on Periscope in early 2015 by Michael Morelli Jr. Instantly the idea sounded genius to me! It's sweet potatoes, not a huge financial investment, and a whole food item, so what's to lose? I went out and purchased some sweet potatoes to get me started! I followed several of Michael's recipes and tips with ease! This diet felt right! I felt clean and satiated while following it! I had no expectations, but to my surprise I lost 12 pounds in the first 13 days! I highly recommend following this diet short term and as a lifestyle! The Sweet Potato Diet has forever changed my life!

—MELISSA B., VIRGINIA BEACH, VA

I was first introduced to the Sweet Potato Diet while following Michael on Snapchat. I had always heard about the many health benefits of sweet potatoes, and have loved them since my junior high days, but other than the "sweet potato casserole" version served at Thanksgiving with my family, I was unaware of how to prepare them. Michael introduced me to sweet potatoes with eggs, with chicken, sweet potato toast, sweet potato hash, etc. I've made them a daily ritual in my diet. My father, who had a stroke last year and has type 2 diabetes, has also benefited from my incorporating sweet potatoes into our diets more. I've gained energy, lost body fat, and have never felt better in my entire life. It's an easy, clean, affordable, efficient, and effective carbohydrate! Thank you, Michael!

—DANIELLE P., RANCHO CUCAMONGA, CA

I began following the Sweet Potato Diet before I even truly knew what it was. I was seeing the hashtag #sweetpotatodiet on Instagram a lot and decided to do a little research on the health benefits of sweet potatoes and started incorporating them into my diet a bit more. Well, eventually all of the hashtags led me to the Morellifit page and this is where my true start on the Sweet Potato Diet began! I ordered a Custom Meal Plan from Michael and his team and I have to say it was life changing. Once I began following his plan and eating not only sweet potatoes but everything else he suggested, I began to notice significant changes in both my physical and emotional well being. I had more energy, my skin and hair became healthier, my mind was more clear, my stamina and endurance increased… and this is just to name a few. Although called a diet, I see it as a lifestyle change. A lifestyle change that I intend to continue living!! Thanks for helping me get my life and my health back!

—JESSICA A.

Sweet Potato Diet change my entire perspective about eating, I didn't know that eating sweet potatoes can change my health and my figure. I'm a diabetic and Sweet potatoes are an excellent source of carbohydrates for those with blood sugar problems. These fibrous root vegetables can help regulate blood sugar levels and prevent conditions like insulin resistance. Thank you, Michael, for introducing this amazing diet!!! Sweet Potato Diet rocks!!!

—TJ

The Sweet Potato Diet has been a total game changer when it comes to achieving my health and fitness goals. I was first introduced to the diet when I started my first Custom Meal Plan. I liked sweet potatoes, but when Michael made me aware of the INSANE benefits, sweet potatoes became my favorite carbohydrate source. After incorporating sweet potatoes into my regular diet, I was able to gain over 15 pounds of lean muscle while maintaining 8% body fat. Not only has the Sweet Potato Diet helped me with my fitness goals, I truly believe that there are incredible long term benefits of choosing sweet potatoes over other carb sources. I hope everyone comes to understand the power of the sweet potato.

—GARRETT S.

Since Michael Morelli introduced the Sweet Potato Diet into my life, it has been a total game changer. I lost 5 pounds the first week I tried it and felt more amazing and energized than I ever had before! Michael has provided many different ways to eat sweet potatoes and I had no idea that meal prep could taste so good! This healthy change has helped me reach fitness goals I had no idea were possible.

—CLARISSA W.

The Sweet Potato Diet has done marvelous things in my life. Before starting with this diet I used to worry about every single calorie I consumed. I calculated everything, including non-starchy vegetables. When I bought my first meal plan from Michael, I was a little bit skeptical and afraid that I would gain all my fat back. I was supposed to eat six times a day, when I was used to eating 2-3 times per day. After a few months following the diet, I was so surprised to see that even though I had gained muscle mass, my body fat kept melting! This diet has changed my life not only because I get to eat without fear but also because I have the freedom to eat the foods I love and enjoy! Thank you so much Michael and your Sweet Potato Diet. My life has changed forever!

—ANDRES C.

The Sweet Potato Diet, along with a new mindset, has helped me throughout my fitness journey and I'm just getting started. Before I was introduced to #sweetpotatoediet I would spent lots of money on groceries; about $300 a month! I didn't know what I should be eating so I tried to get everything that was there. Truth is I was throwing my money in the trash because of the amount that went bad and had to throw away. I literally started losing belief and was just wasting money. I would lose and gain because I couldn't afford it or stick to it. Until I was introduced to the Sweet Potato Diet and developed my mindset, I gave it another shot. I got on a Custom Meal Plan and tried the Sweet Potato Diet. I didn't like them at first but after what it did for my body, I started to love them. I dropped 20 pounds in a month and a half! Not only that, but I cut my grocery expenses by more than half than I would spend before. I'm a man in progress, but eating healthy is starting to become a habit and all credit goes to Michael Morelli Jr. for helping me change my routine and become more aware.

—ALEXIS M. S.

A couple summers ago, I was introduced to the Sweet Potato Diet over social media. It was a life changing moment when I first learned of it. I started eating sweet potatoes morning, noon, and night. In the first month, I lost 20 pounds! To this day, I still eat sweet potatoes every day. I have learned how to utilize the diet for my goals, thanks to Morellifit.

—REESE H.

I first encountered the Sweet Potato Diet from Michael through his YouTube channel. I love sweet potatoes, and being from the South it was so easy to incorporate them into my diet. I love that I get to eat sweet potatoes with every meal and don't feel guilty at all. Thanks to Michael and the Morellifit family I am able to reach my weight loss goals.

—SHANEE E.

The Sweet Potato Diet is more than just an eating habit to me, it's a mindset. When I first saw Michael eating sweet potatoes via social media, and how passionate he was about their benefits I knew I had to give them a try. After that moment I was hooked. I now eat them almost every day, and I love the energy I get from them and how they make me feel vs a regular less clean carb. Sweet potatoes really got me into the thought that "hey, I can eat real food and enjoy it, and actually fuel my body!" I owe it all to Mike for getting me hooked. #sweetpotatodiet

—JORY P.

THE
SWEET POTATO
DIET

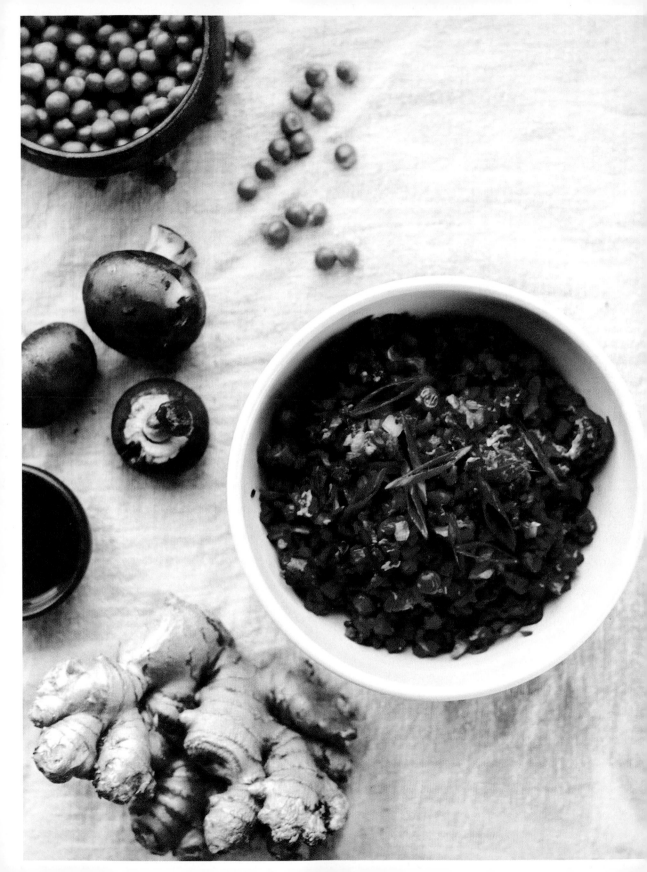

THE
SWEET POTATO
DIET

THE SUPER CARB-CYCLING PROGRAM
to LOSE UP TO 12 POUNDS in 2 WEEKS

MICHAEL MORELLI

Da Capo
LIFE
LONG

PERSEUS BOOKS | HACHETTE BOOK GROUP

Designed by Tabitha Lahr
Set in 10.5 point Minon Pro by Perseus Books

Cataloging-in-Publication data for this book is available from the Library of Congress.

First Da Capo Press edition 2017
ISBN: 978-0-7382-1988-2 (hardcover)
ISBN: 978-0-7382-1989-9 (e-book)

Photography Credit: Constance Higley
Contributing Writer: Rachael Goodrum
Contributing Editor: Lauren Epler

Published by Da Capo Press, an imprint of Perseus Books, LLC, a subsidiary of Hachette Book Group, Inc.
www.dacapopress.com

Note: The information in this book is true and complete to the best of our knowledge. This book is intended only as an informative guide for those wishing to know more about health issues. In no way is this book intended to replace, countermand, or conflict with the advice given to you by your own physician. The ultimate decision concerning care should be made between you and your doctor. We strongly recommend you follow his or her advice. Information in this book is general and is offered with no guarantees on the part of the authors or Da Capo Press. The authors and publisher disclaim all liability in connection with the use of this book.

Da Capo Press books are available at special discounts for bulk purchases in the U.S. by corporations, institutions, and other organizations. For more information, please contact the Special Markets Department at Perseus Books, 2300 Chestnut Street, Suite 200, Philadelphia, PA, 19103, or call (800) 810-4145, ext. 5000, or e-mail special.markets@perseusbooks.com.

10 9 8 7 6 5 4 3 2 1

Thanks to my dad for the constant motivation; even though the words often hurt, they are what drives me.

Thanks to my mother for always bringing new awareness into my life, awareness and feedback that have led me to be the man I am today.

Thanks to my amazing fiancée Amanda for taking care of our family so I could write, pursue, and hack healthy from new angles. Without her, this book, and the transformations of millions of lives, wouldn't be possible.

Thanks to the best kids in the world, Carina and Carmello, for loving me. You have no idea how much that love affects my drive. This is all for you.

Thanks to my amazing community who supports me in everything I do, from supplements and custom nutrition to this very book.

Thank you to my amazing team who make it possible to touch and help millions of people every day. Their authentic love for people is unmatched.

Thanks to Rachael Goodrum for working long hours and being there for me. No matter what, she never said no, she never wavered, and she's a big reason why this book made it to the shelves.

Thanks to Lauren Epler for stepping in and assisting in a major way so we could get this to publish on time.

Thanks to Da Capo for believing in my book despite there being countless books on diet. This, I assure you, changes the game.

Thanks to Nicole, my PR girl, for believing in me and setting up the connection between myself and Sterling Lord, who also happens to be such an amazing group.

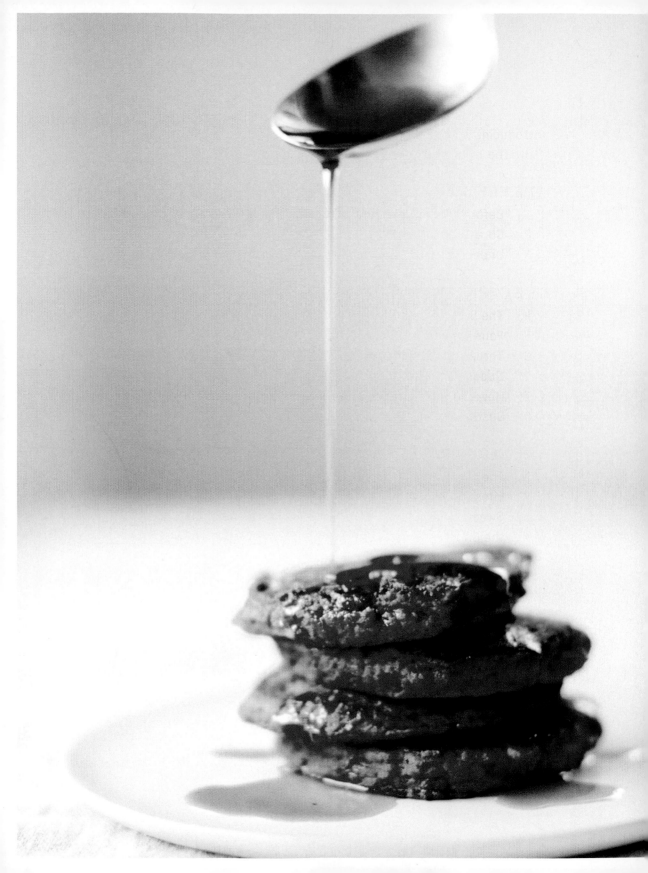

Contents

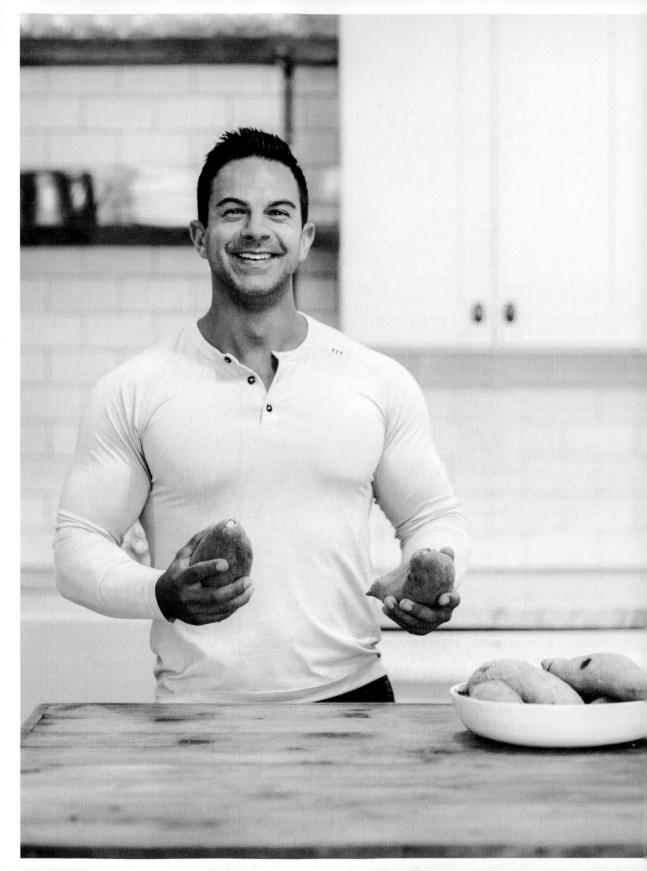

Preface:
Introducing Michael: From Fat to Fit

My story starts over ten years ago. I had been trying to get fit since my early twenties. The problem in my early twenties was that drinking in bars, doing drugs, and chasing girls got in the way of that. And while I was working really hard at the gym, I had absolute crap to show for it. Boy was I out of shape! I was the guy who one week would do cardio because I saw an article in the magazines that said it was best for fat loss, and after a few days (lol) when that didn't work, I would be on to the next. Maybe you can relate? I know after helping hundreds of thousands of people lose fat, that it's a very common cycle people go through. You hear about the latest and greatest diets, supplements, and gadgets, and immediately think it's "your answer." Well, the shiny stuff always got me. I was that guy. I did the fad diets. I tried low carb, no carb, I was on the Atkins and the Zone diets. There were just so many I lost track—it's safe to say I tried everything!

Well, not everything (as you'll read in just a moment). But I had to hit the "rock bottom", a pivotal moment, and I remember it like it was yesterday. I was walking up two flights of stairs, winded, gassed, and out of breath. I finally reached the top (it felt like Mount Everest) with two measly little bags of groceries, one in each hand, winded with a little sweat on the upper lip. I said to myself, "This shit has got to change." At this point I was sick and tired of being sick and tired. It was this pivotal moment, and some news I would receive shortly after, that lit a fire under my ass like I never felt.

At that point, I had no idea where to start. But I remember getting a call that no guy wants to get: She said, "I am pregnant." I said, "Are you sure?" She (my fiancé now) said, "Yes, I am sure." No pressure, heh? News I got at a time when I was down and out. It was bad, and I am not talking about just my health (more on this in a minute).

It's amazing how resourceful you can become in the midst of what at the time felt like a crisis. As far as my health was concerned, remember I had tried everything. Google and I became best friends, and began to sift through the never-ending plethora of diet advice until I stumbled on what the mainstream refers to as the Paleo Diet.

As I read more and more it became almost an obsession. It was the only thing that has ever made sense. If it was going to work, I knew I had to simplify it otherwise I was doomed for failure. I couldn't do the same thing I had done in the past and expect a different outcome—that's just insanity. The baby steps included a more whole foods diet. I slowly—and I repeat, *slowly*—started to replace the processed crap I was eating with whole foods from as close to nature as possible.

I remember the last couple of things to go (haha)! What do you think they were? What would yours be? For me it was cereal and pizza. Damn I love me some Fruity Pebbles! I could polish off a whole pizza and an entire box in one sitting. Looking back: Holy moly, what a chemical shit-storm that was. It was a gradual process that took months and months. The less processed my diet became the better and better I felt. I had more energy—insane amounts actually—and clarity and focus. It was during this time I kicked my alarm, too.

Now that I finally had a good hold on my diet, it was time to take a look at my exercise. Along with my less-processed diet, I started doing what I thought were really cool exercises. I found them online and just started stringing them together. These are exercises that you may have heard of, like burpees, mountain climbers, and planks. More on exercise later, and don't worry, it will be much simpler than that, in fact this diet works like magic even without exercise.

At this time I was very limited, and didn't have the money for a gym membership. As this was all going on I was also going through bankruptcy and divorce (I told you it was real bad!). I was living in a tiny 1,000-square-foot apartment, and all I had access to was a set of dumbbells. It was actually a blessing—remember I had tried the gym before and failed over and over again...

Are you ready? Get this! Just 113 days later, I was able to go from 24% body fat down to 8%, I dropped 27 pounds of fat, and saw my abs for the first time in my life. It was like the fat melted off my body as I witnessed it in real time.

At this time, believe it or not, I had what many refer to as a spiritual awakening. One of my very best friends, and someone I still admire, handed me a Bible. His name was David Olson. It was a little green Bible with my name in it and it had a suggested reading schedule.

I wasted no time. I started reading it every day. You see, David was the kind of guy I wanted to be like. Always positive, caring, sympathetic, and most of all, willing and ready to serve. He had something special and it wasn't money, which I had thought for the longest time equated to happiness. I was, and still am to this day, hungry for growth. Would you believe I made flash cards with biblical verses and started to memorize them?

Four months passed by and all of the growing began to compound, people started to notice me. It felt so good, especially for someone that always craved his dad's approval. Looking back, through all of the client work I have done, I have realized that validation is something that makes us all feel good. I also will always remember my family saying all sorts of positive things. I even remember this girl at a coffee shop I went to regularly noticing my progress. Back then it was called Alterra, it since has been changed to Colectivo. Talk about motivation! There is no better motivation than being noticed and acknowledged for your accomplishments.

Even with all of this very gratifying success, I had a couple big clouds looming. I knew I had to get on the other side of the divorce and bankruptcy in order to really make some serious strides, because what it was doing to my mindset at times was very much holding me back—I could just feel it.

I needed more motivation than just a nice set of abs, so I dug deep in search of something more meaningful than looks or success. Something that could provide me with that lasting motivation, a motivation I could wake up and think of every day. Needless to say it was my little girl Carina Marie. The biggest blessing my life has ever seen. Words can't explain what this little girl has taught me in the four short years she's been in my life.

You see, she deserved a good life. I remember holding her (I was the very first one) like it was yesterday, looking into her eyes (tears filled mine up), and I remember saying to her, "Daddy will not ever fail you." And from that moment on I get a reminder every morning at 7 A.M. and it reads, "You're doing this for your kids," because since then we had Carmello, our little man.

So my quest for knowledge began. I read and read and read. I studied everything from paleo, vegan, IIFYM, carb cycling, and blood/DNA type diets. You name it, I read and studied it. I was hungry (pun intended) and always learning, and that hasn't stopped ever since.

Through all this hunger, a passion had been formulated. I realized my passion was to help others realize their full potential so they, too, could live happier, healthier, more productive lives.

This was all well and good, but I knew if anyone was going to take me seriously, I needed more than just a nice six-pack and a good story. I needed some credibility to go along with it. And so over the next six months I completed a total of five certifications: CPT-ISSA, RKC, CF-L1, OPT, and CrossCore. Today I have a total of six with a certificate in Neural Linguistic Programming (NLP), believe it or not this is the one that allows me to help people break through the mental barriers that we all face from time to time.

Talk about cruising, that was me! My brain, my body, my spirit. I remember fist-pumping through the house saying to myself, "Look out world." Haha! At the time I had absolutely no idea what that meant. I know now that I needed to capture America's attention somehow, someway. And with all of the social media channels sounds easy, right?

But it wasn't. There were thousands of stories just like mine competing for the world's attention. I had to think, what made me any different? At the time I didn't know. But what I did know was that my daughter, only months old, needed me and quitting was not an option. She was depending on me.

So I knew it was time. It was time to put myself out there. I remember my very first video about three years ago (it's still on YouTube). No one was watching, I mean no one. I didn't have even 100 subscribers. I remember being in my mother's basement, bankruptcy finally behind me. It wasn't fun. Imagine being on your own for over a decade and having to move back in with your mom in your thirties, with a newborn and a fiancée.

I will never forget the day. I finally made the commitment in my mind. I set up my iPhone and walked in front nervous as all hell. If you watch that video (and I hope you do) you'll see me rocking back and forth, so much that I probably left a groove in the floor. Haha! Fun times for sure! Lots and lots of retakes and videos later I found a new confidence in myself, one that surely I never knew I had. From that point on it just got easier, now you can't keep me from getting in front of the camera, I love it! From my daily live streams, to the weekly YouTube videos, with daily Snapchat and Instagram posts, you'd think I would have a couple clones!

It's so surreal now that I have such an amazing community that allows me the privilege of sharing my journey. I remember back a few short years ago, months and months went by when no one was listening. I remember for what seemed like forever, I had no subscribers, as in zero!

But then along came Instagram, and I saw lots and lots of action happening, so I quickly started posting daily; multiple times a day in fact. I remember at one point, waking up a couple times through the night so my followers in other parts of the country would see my content. I did this for over a year. My mother thought I was crazy, and poor Amanda. I remember waking her up on several occasions, as if taking care of our newborn wasn't enough. Looking back, I realize just how lucky I am to have such a cheerleader in my corner.

Fast forward just twenty-four months and I have a best-selling program called HIIT MAX™ with over 150,000 copies sold by May 2015. I also have a newsletter with over 300,000 active subscribers and millions of followers all over the world.

Today, just a year later, we are a full-fledged health and wellness company providing custom nutrition and training solutions and some of the cleanest supplements on the market. We have served over 200,000 people through direct sales of products, programs, and services. We have clients on every continent and look forward to serving even more. We also have a very active blog (www.morellifit.com) that's updated with new cutting-edge nutrition and training advice a couple times per week. The daily unique visitors are growing and nothing brings a big smile to my face more than an active, growing community of like-minded individuals who share a passion to live their best.

I chalk up this early success to a couple of key factors: transparency and trust. I have never recommended or put my name on something that I didn't feel was the absolute best. As you read the chapters of this book, it's important to know that I am right there with you, eating sweet potatoes, enjoying the benefits and the results that this lifestyle offers. My entire family eats them as our main carb source, even my kids follow the Sweet Potato Diet, we are all in!

Since my mother's basement, the mission has been: "Let's get fit together." It's through this mission that comes a vision to create a social revolution. By using health and fitness as our catalyst, I believe we can foster a community where people continually grow to the next level of awareness. It's in this environment where people will thrive, and live a life full of abundance and fulfillment.

I believe it's the Sweet Potato Diet and its simplification that lends itself to the cultivation of such a group, and I will always look for what will have the biggest impact on the most amount of people. This is why you're holding this book. This is why I live this book each and every day, and this is why this book is the last diet book you'll ever feel the need to buy.

Not only have the principles in this book paved the way for my new lifestyle, they have also changed the lives of thousands of my clients, and I am proud to share it with you now. The Sweet Potato Diet is based on proven results, from people just like you every single day. Here's to your transformation. And always remember to be patient, stay the course, and let's get fit, together.

—Michael Morelli

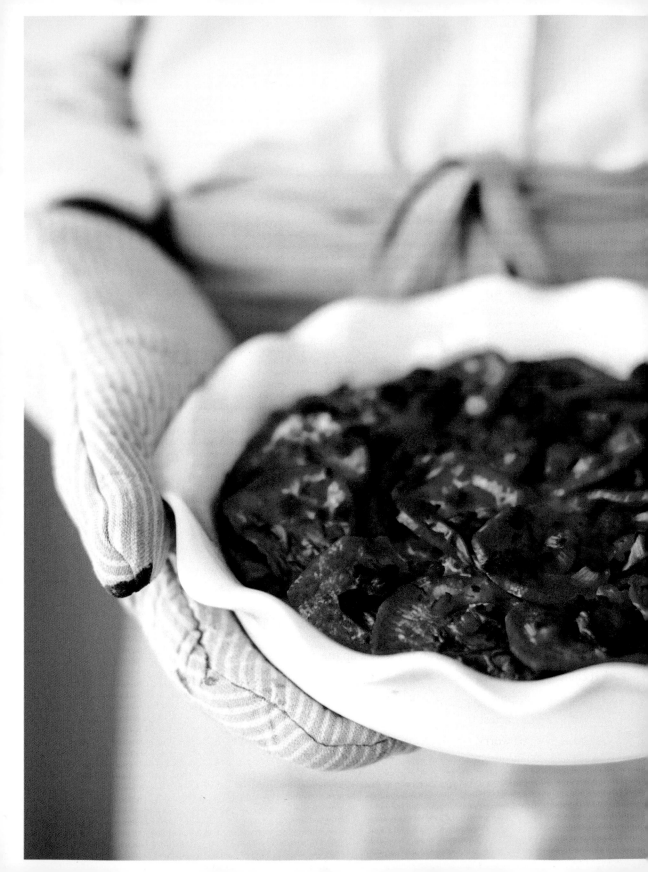

Introduction:
The Truth About Carbs

Why The Sweet Potato Diet Is Different

Carb cycling the Sweet Potato Diet way is a simple yet powerful 7-day eating schedule that harnesses the power of the sweet potato to ignite fat-loss, increase energy, and keep you fuller longer. This means less cravings, keeping you on track for some of the most rapid fat loss you've ever experienced, and the best part is you'll never feel deprived because there are so many tasty recipes to choose from.

Let's face it, the reason so many people fail is because they get impatient, they just don't see results as fast as they would like, or sometimes not at all. The Sweet Potato Diet is unlike any diet I have ever seen (and I've seen and even tried a ton), in that it acts fast creating some early momentum that allows people to gain confidence and control. It's very likely you will see some amazing body composition changes in just the first 7 days. The amazing macro profile of the Sweet Potato has an unforeseen ability to rev-up the metabolism without creating insulin spikes that cause the usual weight gain you've likely experienced with most carbohydrates.

Now add the power of Sweet Potatoes to my crazy (in a good way) carb cycling methodology and you have the fastest fat loss (healthy fat loss of course) ever seen in a diet. If carb cycling is a foreign term don't worry, it sounds way scarier than it actually is. All it means is cycling your carbs from higher to lower (don't worry, we guide you step-by-step) throughout each week. You see, when you manipulate carbs in this way you keep your metabolism guessing (more on this later).

Most other carb cycles only alternate between high and low carb days six times a week, saving the seventh day for the reward meal with very little or no tailoring to each unique person. The Sweet Potato Diet is different and more powerful. It provides you with three different carefully designed 7-day carb cycles (Quick Fire, Activate, or the Accelerated Inferno) all of which combine high-, medium-, low-, and no-carb days for incredible effects and faster results. Plus, the cycle is tailored to exactly what your body needs. I will show you how to create the perfect portions for you specifically, and you won't ever need to count calories or macros (forget that!). Hint: if you can close your fist you can easily do the Sweet Potato Diet. Just remember, one size never fits all (that's why most diets have failed you in the past).

The Sweet Potato Diet will not only have you slimmer in record time, it's unlike most other diets because it will help you keep the weight off—forever! You see that's the ultimate game changer for me. No more rebounds, say goodbye for good, because you'll never meet this fat again.

Why Does the Body Love Carb Cycling So Much?

Carb cycling is really nature's preferred way of getting and staying lean. It:

- Supercharges your metabolism
- Gives you the ability to eat more carbs
- Preserves and promotes lean muscle tissue
- Optimizes fat burning by working with your body
- Maximizes fat loss without losing muscle

Carb Cycling 101 (How Exactly Does It Work?)

When you restrict carbohydrates for an extended period, you lose fat and, in a lot of cases, water weight. But it's not all good news: the longer you deprive your body of carbohydrates, the lower your metabolism can fall.

However, when used correctly, taking carbs out of your nutrient intake for a day is a very effective way of teaching the body to be metabolically flexible. In other words, it gives the body opportunities to use fat for fuel when it needs to on days where there are no carbs.

The trouble with the Standard American Diet is that the body is never given a chance to burn fat because it is so laden with carbohydrates 24 hours a day, 7 days a week, 365 days a year! When was the last time you actually gave your body the chance to burn some fat for a change? Well, using the Sweet Potato Diet will do exactly that for you; it will teach your body to burn fat when it needs to, effortlessly.

That's why using carbohydrates at the right time, on the right days will ensure optimum fat burning without the risk of reducing metabolism. Pretty neat, huh? The Sweet Potato Diet uses a super smart, step-by-step approach to eating the carbs you love. This not only works with your body (we'll teach you), it stays one step ahead of it.

This diet never deprives your body of carbohydrates long enough to allow your metabolism to slow down. The high-carb days are designed to increase your metabolism and prime your body to burn fat on the lower- or no-carb days. On these days, your body switches from burning carbohydrates to catabolic fat burning, actually burning its own stored fat and using it for fuel. Pretty smart, huh?

High-Carb Days Actually Burn Body Fat

A traditional low-carb diet keeps your carbohydrate intake relatively low (below 50g/day) for extended periods of time, then when you attempt to reintroduce carbs, you blow up like a blimp. There's a much better way to drop your carbs, and that's through a cycling format.

You're going to be introducing high-carb days at least twice each week. Your body won't have a chance to adapt to the lower-carb/calorie days, no matter how long you use these cycles for. That's the beauty of carb cycling. We are literally shocking your metabolism into using fat for energy, and the body never gets a chance to get complacent or adapt. No more plateaus and no more frustration ever again. Instead you get ongoing, effective fat loss that lasts, by working with your body's natural systems.

And that's the greatest advantage of carb cycling and the power of your body when you work with it, and not against it. You are literally setting up an inferno in your body, creating a fat-burning furnace, which will sustain a more efficient metabolism for life.

Fad Diets and Water Weight?

Weight loss adverts do it all the time—use outrageous fat loss claims such as, "Lose 20 pounds in 2 weeks." Sounds great. Until you look at the truth behind the hype.

Sure, it might be possible to achieve these results, but what these programs don't reveal is that most of the weight loss comes from dropping water, not actual fat. And they never, ever (at least in my experience), set you up to succeed long-term.

If you lose mostly water weight, what happens when you start eating normally? I mean, you cannot succumb to the "fad diet" lifestyle forever. The water returns and, more often than not, so does the weight. And, FYI, the reality is that your body weight can fluctuate up to 5 or so pounds every day depending on the food consumed, your water intake, hormones (especially women), and your activity level.

That's why it's important to focus on what really matters: fat loss, energy, real food, activity that you love, and living a sustainable lifestyle, just like the four million (and counting) people who are following me on various social media platforms. They're fed up with the diet and fitness industry's promises, and so am I. It's about time for some real answers, heh?

The Sweet Potato Promise

The Sweet Potato Diet promises that you can lose up to 12 pounds of actual body fat (not muscle or water weight) in the first two weeks, and continue dropping body fat over the next few months, and maintain it with minimal exercise.

You'll feel good, have more energy, and experience true lasting weight loss while regaining your health and vitality.

Do I Need to Work Out on the Sweet Potato Diet?

If you can lose fat without much exercise at all, why does the Sweet Potato Diet program ask you to exercise? And why do I absolutely love working out as an integral part of my life?

While it's true that you'll certainly lose plenty of fat on this diet with minimal exercise, it's still important that you stay active for a healthy lifestyle. If you look at those in the later years of life, it's clear that those who have done some exercise are far better off and live a better quality of life. Exercise is also important for emotional and mental wellness, which are critical for a happier, healthier, more productive life.

To get the absolute most out of the Sweet Potato Diet, it's important to be active at least a few days per week. But here's the best part, you get choose the type of exercise. I want you to choose something you love, and just in case I will also give you some recommendations later in the book. Do you want to know what the very best form of exercise for fat loss is? Here's a little secret. Are you ready?

The best form of exercise FOR YOU is the activity you like doing most. Yep, that's it. Find an activity or workout you love and you'll continue to do it because you enjoy it!

Beginner? Don't worry, there's a section on exercise for those who don't regularly work out. You might like to start with a simple activity such as brisk walking (even right in front of your TV) for just a few minutes a day. Believe it or not, I start all of my private clients who haven't exercised in a long time this way and it works every time! You see, it shows you how to build in tiny new habits and eventually those habits become second nature. You'll find it fun and invigorating and may even look to incorporate other exercises like light jogging, rowing, swimming, biking, or kayaking, or your favorite sport for 5–30 minutes a day. Even though these activities aren't too demanding, they're proven to build health, strength, and endurance…and of course, contribute in a major way to fat loss. Another couple of tricks I use to burn extra calories are parking further away; I always park in the last few spots and walk, and always take the stairs when there's an option. You'd be surprised at how many extra calories you burn over the course of the week by making these simple adjustments, not to mention the great benefits to your overall health.

Intermediate or advanced? You could opt for high intensity interval training (HIIT) or strength training (which are my preferences). The section later in the book on incorporating your workouts into the Sweet Potato Diet will help you get the most out of both the carb cycle and your current fitness routine. I also have loads of fitness tips and workouts I've put together on our YouTube Channel.

Remember, the Promises You're Used to Hearing from the Diet Industry Are All Lies

As we dig deeper, please remember one very important thing: I pledge to only give you the truth. Even though it may not always be what you want to hear, it's been the backbone of my entire business since I started three short years ago in my mom's basement. If you know me from my work in the industry, you'd be nodding your head with confidence right now because transparency and truth is what I'm known for.

This book is going to set you up for long-term success, fast fat loss, and a sustainable lifestyle, so you can live happier, healthier, and be more productive and vibrant every day.

Fad diets don't work long-term; they are sexy but they don't work, and that's just the fuel I needed to write this book.

Remember one very important thing as we move forward:

Healthy and sustainable weight loss is only achieved when you lose body fat and maintain lean body mass (muscle).

The Unnoticeable Differences Are Actually the Key

When fat loss occurs, the differences in your body are visible. But there are other major benefits to shedding unwanted fat the healthy way, too. You've got so much more to look forward to, just wait and trust me, it feels amazing!

Your family and friends will quickly begin to notice the physical changes, and that's a great first step (because we're pretty harsh critics of our own bodies).

Your clothes will fit better, you'll be able to get back into old favorites, and may even need to go clothes shopping (haha fun!).

You're also going to feel better than you ever thought possible and experience:

- Increased energy and no afternoon crashes
- Wake up feeling rested and refreshed
- Experience better moods and fewer swings
- Curb cravings and deal with them better
- Be strong and more confident in everyday life

The Sweet Potato Diet Has Everything You Need and a Bag of Chips

Ok, so we don't want to be eating chips, unless they're sweet potato chips—haha, no really, there are some chips you can eat on this diet. They are made by Jackson's Honest, and get this, the only ingredients are sweet potatoes, coconut oil, and a little sea salt.

The Sweet Potato Diet you have in your hands contains everything you need to get started on your new journey and transformation. You don't need to purchase anything else. This is it!

All the fluff has been removed. And I've made it very easy to follow. All you need to do is to be patient, follow the blueprint, and stay the course. We have divided your journey into two phases, and this is so you can navigate through it and refer back with ease. This way you can go back and reference various points throughout your entire journey.

And I'm right here to support you. I mean it: if you need to contact me, please don't hesitate. You can reach me on Twitter @morellifit (and please do!)—I want you to succeed!

Introducing the Sweet Potato

By now it should be obvious that the sweet potato is the center of this diet. But why?

Most of the world views the sweet potato as just another potato. But there is more to the sweet potato than meets the eye. Aside from not having a strong relation to the regular white potato, the nutrients and benefits of this vegetable make it a powerhouse of health. Its journey around the world and throughout history is a vast one, and all of these things make it the perfect choice to center the carb cycle around.

GENERAL BIOLOGY

The scientific name for the sweet potato is "Ipomoea batatas." Ipomoea is derived from several Greek words that translate to "resembling bindweed," a name that most likely comes from the fact that the sweet potato has a habit of twining and growing like the bindweed itself. The word "batatas" comes from the Tanino (Central American) language, stemming from the word "batata," meaning potato. This name most likely came over with the Spaniards, who brought the sweet potato back with them from Central America.

The sweet potato, although a potato, is not a close relative of the more common white potato. White potatoes, or common potatoes, are tubers and are more closely related to eggplants, hot peppers, and tomatoes. The sweet potato, on the other hand, is from the Morning Glory plant family and instead is a vine, which has thick roots for storing water and nutrients. The sweet potato is the thick root of this plant.

The sweet potato is also different than the yam. Although these two are sometimes confused, they are not the same plant, nor are they from the same family. Yams originated in West Africa, unlike sweet potatoes, whose origins go back to Central America. Both are grown in tropical regions, but the yam is a coarse and hairy root and the sweet potato is smoother with a thinner skin. The yam is not grown anywhere in the United States. The USDA requires any potato labeled "yam" to also be labeled as a sweet potato because it is not truly a yam.

NUTRITION POWER OF THE SWEET POTATO

NUTRITIONS	Amount per serving	% daily value
Saturated Fat	0 g	0%
Cholesterol	0 mg	0%
Sodium	41 mg	2%
Total Carbohydrate	24 g	8%
Dietary Fiber	4 g	15%
Sugars	7 g	--
Protein	2 g	--
VITAMINS		
Vitamin A	21907 IU	438%
Vitamin C	22.3 mg	37%
Vitamin D	--	--
Vitamin E (Alpha Tocopherol)	0.8 mg	4%
Vitamin K	2.6 mcg	3%
Thiamin	0.1 mg	8%
Ribloflavin	0.1 mg	7%
Niacin	1.7 mg	8%
Vitamin B6	0.3 mg	16%
Folate	6.8 mcg	2%
Vitamin B12	0.0 mcg	0%
Pantothenic Acid	1.0 mg	10%
Choline	14.9	--
Betaine	39.4	--
MINERALS		
Calcium	43.3 mg	4%
Iron	0.8 mg	4%
Magnesium	30.8 mg	8%
Phosphorus	61.6 mg	6%
Potassium	541 mg	15%
Sodium	41.0 mg	2%
Zinc	0.4 mg	2%
Copper	0.2 mg	9%
Manganese	0.6 mg	28%
Selenium	0.2 mcg	0%
Fluoride	--	--

HEALTH BENEFITS OF THE SWEET POTATO

The health benefits of sweet potatoes are immense, which is why this root is so widely cultivated, not only for its reliable growth, but also for its nutritional power. This root is high in fiber and aids in digestion and colon health. Its low glycemic index can help stabilize blood sugar, which can not only aid in insulin response, but can also be helpful to diabetics, whose blood sugar is a concern when eating foods that can spike blood sugar levels. This food provides plenty of long-term energy because it's a complex carb that can be digested more slowly over time.

The sweet potato's anti-inflammatory properties come from being rich in vitamin A and carotenoids. These help fight inflammation in the body, which can often lead to autoimmune disorders, even arthritis, and cancer. Additionally, carotenoids are antioxidants that can help fight free radicals in the body that have been known to cause cancer.

On top of these amazing properties, the sweet potato can help aid in weight loss. High fiber foods are great to keep you full and can help increase satiation after eating. Plus, being full on such a nutrient-dense food makes sure that not only are fewer calories consumed, but the calories are rich in nutrients. The blood stabilization effects from the sweet potato help with insulin response, which can prevent fat storage over time. This is why sweet potatoes are the perfect choice when choosing the best carbohydrate for carb cycling. Aside from being nutrient rich, the history of the sweet potato is also rich and tells the story of a vegetable that has sustained life for many nations.

THE SWEET POTATO IN NORTH AMERICA

The English brought the sweet potato to North America, where it has enjoyed a very opulent history. By 1796, the sweet potato had appeared in Amelia Simmons's cookbook, *American Cookery,* which is considered to be the first cookbook in the country. In 1840, the cookbook *Directions for Cooker,* by Eliza Leslie, included several recipes for sweet potatoes. By 1936, George Washington Carver published his *How the Farmer Can Save His Sweet Potatoes and Ways of Preparing Them for the Table,* which included over thirty ways of preparing the sweet potato.

The story of how the sweet potato became so popular in the United States is a story of how slavery made this "poor food" an American staple. In colonial America, as far back as 1648, the early colonists in Virginia were growing sweet potatoes as a crop to live on. As colonists moved further into the continent, so did the sweet potato. By the time Eliza Leslie published her cookbook there was a traveler who noted that in a poor rural Mississippi town, sweet potatoes were a crop that life in the area depended on.

Even though it was once regarded as a "poor" food for both blacks and whites in the South, the Revolutionary War changed that. It was the sweet potato that was given out in rations during the war to get soldiers through and General Francis Marion of South Carolina held his men over for months on it. But even after that, the sweet potato was mostly used to feed slaves and poor white families. By the time the Civil War broke out in America, the sweet potato was called on again to help feed the masses who were war-torn and out of supplies. It was the sweet potato that helped Southerners from all classes during the war-torn years and kept families nourished while other crops remained scarce.

WHY WE PICKED IT

The sweet potato's extensive history throughout the world, especially in the United States, makes it not only a healthy and hearty vegetable, but also the perfect root for the Sweet Potato Diet. Carb cycling with the sweet potato makes sense due to the nutrition, the satiating effects, and the overall wellness that it can bring to those who eat it. Simplifying carbohydrates in this diet down to just the sweet potato creates a versatile, widely available, and well-rounded source of nutrition for those who carb cycle for weight loss and overall health.

Presenting: The Sweet Potato Diet

A few years ago, I hated sweet potatoes. I could not stand them. My aunt would make sweet potatoes with marshmallows and nuts on top, and even as sweet as that made them, I still hated them. But for those who know me now, I literally have sweet potatoes morning, noon, and night. I love them for the taste now, as well as for all of the health benefits. I smile every time I eat them because I know I couldn't be eating a better carb. Not only that, sweet potatoes keep my fat storage at bay due to their low glycemic load which keeps insulin to a minimum. They are also loaded with beta-carotene and all sorts of other vitamins and nutrients making them the perfect carbohydrate for fat loss and overall health and wellness.

We have seen amazing results from people who remove all of the other carbohydrates from their diet and replace them with sweet potatoes. From processed carbohydrates like donuts and Twinkies, to less refined carbs like rice and whole grain bread, we replace all of these with sweet potatoes. We asked clients to replace them without counting or measuring. And just from that, they are seeing a significant amount of fat loss. Take it one step further and put this into a carb cycle, we then can manipulate your macros even further, which shocks your body into continued fat loss.

What most people don't understand about weight loss is that it is not just cutting calories. Calorie-cutting diets, where you don't have more than 1,000 calories a day to function, are getting increasingly popular. Initially this leads to weight loss, so it might seem like a good way to keep losing weight. Sometimes even doctors will tell you that's the way to go, just slash the calories below your TDEE (total daily energy expenditure) and you're set. No way, José! Because as we know, your metabolism always adapts to the conditions you impose on it, so before you know it, you flatline and hit a major plateau and when you flatline on 1,000 calories a day, it's terrible for your body.

Your thyroid goes, your metabolism is shot, you're overweight, and you're getting sicker and sicker. You go back to your doctor who is supposed to be helping you get better and instead you get worse. And instead of educating patients on why they are sick and trying to help them prevent it, they usually just prescribe the most incentivized medications. Oftentimes, these medicines just put a Band-Aid on the bigger problem of poor nutrition and lack of information. This is a vicious cycle that a majority of society lives in and the reason why obesity and heart disease are on the rise, along with prescription medication.

Patients continue to eat poorly and become dependent on these medicines. The pharmaceutical industry is a business. In the US alone, it is a 300-billion-dollar market that is on track to reach 400 billion in just three short years (World Health Organization, 2015). When is enough going to be enough and who is going to step up and be held accountable for this health crisis? Leaders in the fitness industry need to step up and do their role to make an honest impact and help people change their lives.

This is the premise behind the Sweet Potato Diet. That is why we use sweet potatoes, an inexpensive but nutrient dense food that is widely available, and we make it so damn simple to work into any lifestyle. We not only help people make changes, they become informed through our social media channels, where we really work hard to be accessible. Our entire foundation has been built on integrity, and it's easy to see because of how transparent we are in everything we do. We want you to follow this lifestyle, get healthy, and live long and vibrantly.

That is where carb cycling comes into play the sweet potato way. We use carb cycling, with sweet potatoes, to shock the metabolism so it never has the opportunity to adapt to the conditions we impose. You'll never flatline, you'll continue to drop body fat, and you'll enjoy some major health benefits in the process. That's a win–win–win in my book!

And, that's doing it all with enough calories to function and be active throughout the day. The Sweet Potato diet takes a carb cycling approach, with some additional details, and really simplifies it. It's bare bones, using a fist, a palm, or fingertips to measure the various macronutrients. And it requires just a sweet potato for carbohydrates to ignite fat loss.

We simplified our diet because people far too often get fixated on the details and that leads to major procrastination, anxiety, and ultimately, failure. Our brains tend to overthink everything and I can't remember what book I read it in, but complexity is the enemy of execution.

We don't want you to read this and feel stuck. This is the unstuck, and the last diet book you will ever have to read. It's sustainable, so feel free to use and reference it forever. It will undoubtedly get you to your ideal body weight. Once you have hit your body weight goal you can use it to guide you in managing your weight pretty effortlessly from that point on.

This book is designed to be fun and entertaining. It is the story of a man and his infamous sweet potatoes sweeping the nation. In this book, you can find recipes and the transformations of other people who have gone before you. It's your complete step-by-step blueprint to carb cycling. Not only is the Sweet Potato Diet fun and easy to follow, you'll learn a little bit about the science behind this incredible, delicious tuber.

I believe in carb cycling wholeheartedly and that's why I have been using it extensively in my own life, as well as teaching hundreds of thousands of other people how to incorporate it into their lives. In my opinion, it's one of the only diets you can do forever and not get bored or discouraged.

I know, from personal experience, it promotes sustainable weight loss and long-term health. Since your body never has the opportunity to adjust, you will never hit another plateau or flatline ever again.

I have seen this diet work for people of all shapes, sizes, and body types. It doesn't matter if you have a slow metabolism or have failed in the past—the Sweet Potato Diet is your solution. Thank you for choosing my book and for giving me the opportunity to join you on this amazing fitness journey.

Two Essential Phases of the Sweet Potato Diet

The Sweet Potato Diet is no ordinary diet because it completely simplifies eating. It follows distinct phases to really skyrocket your success:

- Two phases
- Three special cycle options
- Four different carb days

Two Phases

For optimal results, it's critical that you follow the two phase protocol. Each phase serves an important purpose and you just won't get the same results without them both.

THE PREP PHASE (PHASE 1)

For seven days (while you're reading this book) all you'll do is replace all of your carbohydrates in your diet with sweet potatoes. This is bread, pastas, baked goods, and any grains. It also includes donuts, Ho Ho's, Twinkies, bagels, and chips (unless they are Jackson's Honest Sweet Potato Chips). And if you have any questions about what qualifies as a carbohydrate, I will answer them in the next few chapters.

This phase is designed to jump-start your fat loss and set you up for success in Phase 2. You'll discover everything you need to know to immediately **begin losing weight** and keep it off.

The Prep Phase requires the completion of seven successful days of eating just sweet potatoes as your carbs, as well as understanding the fundamentals in these chapters:

- **CHAPTER 1:** Before You Get Started
- **CHAPTER 2:** Core Eating Principles
- **CHAPTER 3:** Understanding Super Carbs and Essential Nutrition

This is all fundamental to your success, laying down a solid foundation for you to:

- Build the correct eating patterns with proper food choices.
- Get into the habit of healthy eating.
- Begin making smarter choices.
- See the changes in your body.
- Kick-start your sluggish metabolism and weight loss.

Focus on choosing whole foods. Eliminate all processed and refined foods and follow my "90/10 rule"—eat clean 90% of the time, and have a little fun 10% of the time. So that means 1 out of every 10 meals can be whatever you choose, it's your reward meal. Eat and enjoy guilt-free, you earned it, and it's built into the blueprint.

During this phase, you just need to swap in sweet potatoes, but do not worry about measuring or carb cycling just yet. And only eat from the list of approved foods (see pages 143–145—don't worry, there's hundreds of choices), and just make sure to keep your carbs limited to sweet potatoes. In the grocery guide you will see there are healthy carb options, but for right now you don't need to worry about those—it's all about the sweet potato at this point.

If you get off track during this phase, be kind to yourself. Don't beat yourself up about it. Just get back on track as soon as possible.

Rome wasn't built in a day, so cliché, I know, but it's the truth. You didn't put on all that weight overnight, how could you possibly lose it that fast. You can't. However, now you have a blueprint that works, and all you need to do is follow it. Remember, it takes time to build new habits. I know once you complete 7 full days (consecutively) of eating just sweet potatoes and food from the healthy grocery guide, that you'll be ready for Phase 2. Just remember to stick with it, no matter how many times you have to restart. You'll form powerful habits which are going to serve you for a lifetime—my promise!

With this solid foundation, you'll enter Phase 2, The Carb Cycle. The people who complete the prep virtually guarantee themselves **at least a few pounds of fat loss during the first 7 days of the Prep Phase. I have seen as much as 12 pounds of fat loss in 7 days. Crazy, heh?!** Remember, you must complete 7 full days before starting on the Carb Cycling Phase.

Remember to use your *Meal Planner/Food Journal, Grocery Lists, and Recipes.* It's all right here for you.

THE CARB CYCLING PHASE (PHASE 2)

The Carb Cycling phase is designed to help you continue burning fat; here's where you will achieve your first fat loss goal. Keep in mind, we are setting you up for long-term, sustainable results and the Sweet Potato Diet has been specifically designed to help you maintain 100% of your fat loss results.

- **CHAPTER 4:** The Science of Super Carb Cycling
- **CHAPTER 5:** Four Super Carb Days
- **CHAPTER 6:** Three Fat Burning Cycles and Portioning Your Super Carb Cycling Meals
- **CHAPTER 7:** How to Track Results and Read the Signs
- **CHAPTER 8:** Busting Out the Big Guns: The Plateau Breaker

By completing the entire Carb Cycling Phase, you'll put yourself among the men and women who are able to move on with their lives without ever worrying about their weight again.

Before beginning the Carb Cycling Phase (Phase 2), answer the following review questions about Phase 1. If the answers to these questions come quickly and without barriers, you are ready to move on. If not, please be aware of these things as you learn about them later in the book.

- How is your overall food quality?
- Have you been consuming enough protein?
- What is your eating frequency? Is it consistent?
- How much water do you drink each day?
- Are your carb sources in line with what was recommended?
- What types of fats are you using? Are you cooking with coconut oil?
- Do you feel rested when you wake up? How are your energy levels and mood throughout the day?

These questions keep you on track to meet or exceed your fat loss goals. How you answer will say a lot about what you have been able to achieve through implementing the changes and diet introduced in the Prep Phase.

And, if you've successfully completed the Prep Phase, you've already likely shed several pounds or more of fat.

You can stay on the Carb Cycling Phase until you reach your goal weight. After that, you have two choices:

1. Go back to a more moderate carb lifestyle, eating the same quantity of carbs each day of the week using the sweet potato as your carb source 75% of the time or better.

2. Or stay in the Carb Cycling Phase indefinitely. This allows you to continually adjust your carb and calorie intake to maintain your ideal body weight. Personally, I've tried a bunch of different eating plans. And after having carb cycled for the last couple years, I feel it's the best eating lifestyle out there. That's why I'll continue to do it long into the future.

It all comes down to personal preference. However, keep in mind that you can use carb cycling on a long term basis. Just keep making minor tweaks so you continue moving toward your goals.

Whether you use the Carb Cycling Phase for the short-term or the long haul, you'll set yourself up for a lifetime of having a healthier, leaner, and more attractive body 365 days a year…without ever having to diet again.

Knowledge Is Not Power

Knowledge is not power. Applied knowledge with the right effort and intention is power. So do me a favor. Apply the information is this book. You spent money on it, it's not a paperweight, it's your solution to as close to effortless fat loss as I know. When you apply both phases, as well as the rest of the information outlined in this book, rest assured your results are just around the corner—just be patient enough to see them because they are coming, you have my word!

Be patient, stay the course, and let's get fit together.

PART 1:
THE PREP PHASE

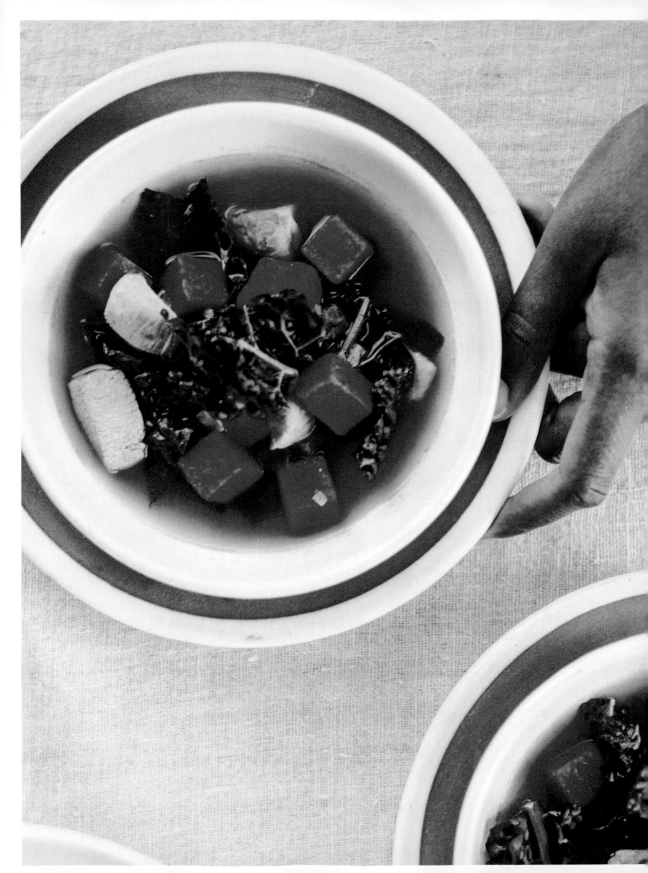

CHAPTER 1:

Before You Get Started

Beat the Odds

According to research published by the *Journal of the American Medical Association,* over one-third (34.9%) of the adults in the US are defined as obese, or having a Body Mass Index (BMI) that is 30 or above. Our waist size isn't the only thing to suffer: obesity hits our wallets hard, too, with additional medical costs on the rise.

We are getting fatter AND poorer. This downward spiral makes a lot of people feel there is no way out.

But there is a solution. The answer slams the brakes on the downward spiral and gives you the power to reverse the trend. You'll be leaner, lighter, and healthier. You'll regain control of your weight, eating habits, and happiness. And you'll save money, too.

To get started on any journey, you need to know where you are right now.

For fat loss, this means calculating your BMI (body mass index).

Calculating Your BMI

Your BMI number uses your height and weight to give you a risk factor for certain serious medical conditions (which can drive your medical cost upwards—and your health downwards).

Here are BMI numbers for a 5' 4" female:

WEIGHT	BMI	THIS MEANS YOU ARE...
Under 110 pounds	Under 18.5	Underweight
110 to 144 pounds	18.5 to 24.9	At a healthy weight
145 to 173 pounds	25 to 29.9	Overweight
174 to 232 pounds	30 to 39.9	Obese
Over 232 pounds	40 and up	Morbidly obese

For a 5' 8" male:

WEIGHT	BMI	THIS MEANS YOU ARE...
Under 125 pounds	Under 18.5	Underweight
125 to 163 pounds	18.5 to 24.9	At a healthy weight
164 to 196 pounds	25 to 29.9	Overweight
197 to 262 pounds	30 to 39.9	Obese
Over 262 pounds	40 and up	Morbidly obese

To calculate *your own BMI,* just go to the National Heart, Lung, and Blood Institute's website at http://www.nhlbi.nih.gov/health/educational/lose_wt/BMI/bmicalc.htm and enter your height and weight. You'll get an instant result telling you exactly where you are at today's weight.

So you know where you are. And you know where you want to be.

Now…how do you get there?

I struggled with this question for an entire decade. I followed advice from every health "expert" or "guru" that offered it. Unfortunately, none of it worked.

I made it my mission to learn how to lose weight effectively, efficiently, and—most important of all—permanently. Here's what I discovered. True fat loss requires going back to eating whole and natural foods and ditching the processed, mass-produced options we have today. That includes the convenient "health foods" packaged to trick us into thinking they can lead us to real health. Changing our lifestyles and making a commitment to choose health over convenience is the only thing that works.

You CAN Beat the Odds

Listen, you don't have to be a statistic, too. No matter how long you've struggled, or what your family history with weight might be, it doesn't have to be your future.

Follow my results-proven program and you will learn how to drop your excess weight and keep it off for good. The best part is that you will do it without having to restrict and deprive yourself, or constantly feel as if you're fighting off cravings.

I *know* that you can beat the odds and avoid joining the 34.9% of Americans currently defined as obese. And if you are obese, this book is here to help you step out of that statistic and lead a healthy and happy life. Make the decision to lose weight once and for all, and make it right now.

Welcome to your future: the way YOU want it to be.

How Our Diet Went Wrong

When you hear the word "diet," what do you think? Favorite foods that are now off limits? Eating weird foods that taste like cardboard? Cravings that haunt you all day (and sometimes in your sleep)?

The real meaning of the word "diet" is the way we eat. It does not have to mean restriction, deprivation, crazy supplements, or becoming "the weird one" in your social group.

Diet just means nutrition. The way you eat today, your food preferences, your behaviors and habits, and, of course, the food choices you make.

"Diet" has become a very emotional word, used to make us scared and fearful, feeling inadequate and full of self-doubt.

Forget the "diet industry" and reclaim the word diet the way it's designed to be used. Don't let those four little letters D-I-E-T make you uncomfortable. It's just another word for the way you eat.

Hunter-Gatherers Turned Farmers

Time for a quick history lesson. Several major changes over the years altered the way we eat, and had a huge impact on our bodies along the way. Truth is, our foods are not what they once were. Today, much of the problem lies in how our food is grown, harvested, and manufactured.

Our genetics are fundamentally the same as early humans', but our diet is wildly different. Is it any wonder our poor bodies struggle to keep up? Our genes want us to eat like early mankind, yet we stuff our bodies with chemicals, processed foods, and crazy manufactured ingredients which are a world away from their natural origins.

Anthropologists have studied fragments of skeleton found in Tanzania in 2012, thought to be 1.5 million years old, and concluded that mankind was eating meat that long ago.

A study published in the *European Journal of Clinical Nutrition* in 2000 concluded that isotope studies of bone chemistry confirmed Neanderthals were top-level carnivores.

It seems our early ancestors dined on a diet that was 70% meat and fish, with a far greater proportion being seafood than what most people eat today.

And guess what? Those ancestors did not eat grains. Even the most basic forms of cereal and grains were not domesticated until around 8,000 years ago. That's a blink of the eye as far as our genetics (and digestion) is concerned. Even then, quantities were small, as wild grain was sparse.

The methods we use for producing food today are relatively new. Commercial farming, domesticated grain and cereal crops, mass production of manmade products, and highly processed foods have changed our nutrition beyond anything our bodies can recognize at a cellular level.

Stop for a minute and think about what that means for your body. Is it any wonder losing fat has seemed such a challenge?

From Natural to Industrial Food

Even a few hundred years ago, many people still lived off the land in small rural farm communities. They harvested freshly-picked produce and sold hand-raised animals. Today, we are oblivious to the source of most of our food.

World Health Organization statistics show the urban population in 2014 accounted for 54% of the total global population.

So what happened?

In a rush to feed the masses and earn profits, mega corporations took control of most of the world's food production. The focus now is on cheap, highly-processed food designed to have a long shelf life with a heavy dependence on cheap grains, soy, and corn.

Meals are now ready straight out of the box or can and on the plate in minutes, instead of hours. The result? Health problems, weight gain, and even psychological and physiological dependence on these chemically altered foods.

We no longer know where our food comes from or how it's made. Believe me, if you look at the long list of ingredients in processed foods, it is abundantly clear that we don't know half of the ingredients we feed our bodies.

Let's stop this cycle for ourselves and our children.

Let's get back to nature.

The Fat Rush

How many of us grab something quick and convenient when we need to eat? This quick-grab mentality fills our bodies with empty calories, sugar, bad fats, and salt.

And if you don't eat out often, you're not immune. According to a 2013 National Health and Nutrition Examination Survey, nearly two-thirds of the added sugars in foods were consumed at home (67.2%) as well as bad fats and excess salt.

So what's the answer?

The answer is cleaning up our diets, both at home and out, becoming more aware consumers, and simplifying our diets back to the whole foods it once consisted of. A cleaner, healthier diet can reverse health problems, save us money, and help us live a leaner, happier lifestyle. It goes way beyond dropping excess fat weight (although that will happen, too).

We're going to focus on a diet rich in nutrition, such as:

LEAN GRASS-FED MEATS—Grass-fed products (which won't have been treated with hormones) are rich in healthy essential omega-3 and omega-6 fatty acids, but low in the bad fats linked with disease.

FRESH SEAFOOD AND SHELLFISH—Good sources of omega-3 and omega-6 fatty acids, selenium, and vitamins A, C, and E. Focus on smaller fish varieties such as mackerel, sardines, or anchovies for the most benefit without risk of contamination.

FRESH PRODUCE—Buy fruits and vegetables that are grown as close to home as possible and make sure they are organic (to eliminate pesticides and herbicides). Spinach, avocado, kale, cabbage, and asparagus are all high in vitamins and minerals. Great fruits include apples, grapefruit, tomatoes, cantaloupes, and berries.

EGGS—Whole eggs are nutritional powerhouses, packed with protein and high in vitamins A, B6, and B12. Try to buy pasture-raised eggs from hens free to roam on open grassland and eat a natural diet.

NUTS AND SEEDS—Our ancestors seemed to favor hazelnuts, but almonds, cashews, pecans, and walnuts are good, too. Nuts are high in fat, so eat them in moderation. Pumpkin seeds and sunflower seeds are great options for snacking or to add crunch to a meal.

HEALTHY OILS – Deep fried foods should be eliminated from your diet, but if you want to stir fry or sauté vegetables, use a healthy oil like olive, walnut, flaxseed, macadamia, avocado, or coconut. These oils should be unprocessed and unrefined, to make sure you are getting the most out of their nutritional profile. Avoid processed (polyunsaturated) vegetable and seed oils, such as soybean, canola, and corn oil.

These few changes mark the start of your new fat loss lifestyle that will see you shedding pounds and keeping them off, whilst boosting your health and energy.

The 7 Roadblocks to Weight Loss (And How You'll Get Around Them)

If you've ever struggled with weight loss in the past, hit a plateau, or fallen back into destructive food behaviors, you'll recognize at least one item on this list.

I've identified 7 reasons which underpin everyone's struggle to lose weight or keep it off. Men, women, young, old, sporty, or sedentary, it doesn't matter. These 7 reasons can be our downfall.

Be aware of them so you can avoid them. With the Sweet Potato Diet, these roadblocks will barely feel like speed bumps.

1. NOT KNOWING WHAT FOODS TO EAT

Unfortunately, many diet books give very general directions. They might tell you all about fats, proteins, and carbohydrates, but there is never any concrete information about the specific foods themselves.

If you don't know which foods to buy from the grocery store and what needs to be stocked in your kitchen, then you will have a tough time. There is no way around this. Guesswork does not make for a successful fat loss plan.

Later inside this book, you will be given lists of foods, so you will be left with no doubt about what to eat for fat loss. This removes all the confusion from the shopping process.

The grocery store can be intimidating, especially if you don't know where to look or what to ask for. I'll give you a 1-2-3 step-by-step approach. All you have to do is to print off the checklist and shop. It will be like I am right there shopping with you.

2. NOT KNOWING HOW MANY TIMES TO EAT

Do you know how frequently to eat for maximum fat loss? Do you know the one time of day you must avoid eating if you want to lose fat?

These things make a big difference. Meal frequency and timing is important, especially initially as you build in better eating habits. It can make or break you for sure.

Making one small shift in meal frequency will have a major impact on the way your body responds. I know it may sound contradictory, but you've got to eat if you want to lose weight.

3. NOT KNOWING HOW TO COMBINE FOODS

While most people know about the fat-inducing foods and the healthiest foods to eat, most people are never told about combining foods.

Yet this is one of the most important concepts in burning fat. It turns out that there are certain combinations of foods that the body requires to stay lean.

I figured this out after years of trial and error. But have you ever read about it in any "diet guru" book?

The lack of food combination for fat loss is one of the reasons generic "low fat" or "low carb" diets do not work. They don't allow the body the combinations of foods that it needs to burn fat and stay healthy. You cannot eliminate an entire macronutrient without your body fighting back.

4. OBSESSION WITH COUNTING CALORIES

Most people lose interest in a diet program as soon as they find out that they need to count calories and measure their food.

Let's be real: Most people simply don't have the time to count every crumb that they consume. It's just unrealistic.

With the Sweet Potato Diet, you need to have a general understanding of calories (which I'll give you), but you don't need to count them up. Why? Because we're eating real, whole foods which our bodies instinctively know how to process.

I'll also show you how to use the simple "palm" approach to portion control. One serving of protein is the size of your flat palm, one serving of carbohydrates is the size of your fist, and a fat serving is the size of your thumb. How easy is that?

You're going to learn something important—how to eat until you are about 70% full. You will soon get used to the natural feeling that your body gives you when you've had enough to eat.

5. BEING OVERWHELMED BY INFORMATION

Information overload cripples dieters.

I know this from personal experience. There is so much conflicting and inaccurate information on the Internet, it's hard to know who to trust or where to start.

Conflicting information leads to procrastination.

With the Sweet Potato Diet, you get real, up-front information and a plan that can be followed from day one. No more guesswork, doubt, or procrastination. Just results.

6. NOT HAVING ENOUGH TIME TO PREPARE MEALS

What *The Sweet Potato Diet* will show you is that even the busiest parent or most stressed executive can prepare healthy, delicious meals that lead to fat loss. No complicated recipes and no need to spend hours in the kitchen. It all comes down to staying prepared by prepping your food in advance, so you can grab and go when you need to.

The importance of food prep is HUGE. I'll teach you how and give you tools that no one else ever talks about.

7. BELIEVING YOUR BODY IS UNABLE TO LOSE WEIGHT

I spoke earlier about the diet industry keeping us in a state of fear and inadequacy. Many people have formed the belief that they cannot achieve the body of their dreams. They think they are destined to be heavy, unhealthy, and overweight.

The problem isn't a lack of effort or willpower. The problem is the information and advice that pervades the modern diet industry.

Before we move on, I want you to think about one point:

The human body always responds to the same stimulus, regardless of the personal characteristics and beliefs in your brain.

Your body is a series of systems and genes.

Once you start eating properly, it will respond in the way it's been designed to. Your metabolism shifts, and you become a fat-burning machine.

Avoid the Most Damaging Weight Loss Myths Most People Believe

If you're going to be a Sweet Potato Diet success story, you need to know about the most commonly held myths that keep millions of men and women fat—and they don't even know it.

Simply believing one of these shocking myths can totally derail your fat loss, even with the power of the Sweet Potato Diet.

It's crucial that we get these out of the way before you start. You need to know that:

- You can lose weight without starvation diets, constant cravings, and hours of endless cardio.
- A fat loss diet does not have to affect your relationships and social life.
- You don't need low-fat diets, no-carb diets, Atkins, Zone, or any other celebrity-endorsed diets or pills.

Those diet myths offer tempting promises, but they deliver nothing but poor health and eventually weight gain because they are just aren't sustainable.

Let's have some fun by dismissing the most widespread, commonly believed myths that are just waiting to sabotage your weight-loss success.

All carbs are bad	Nope. There are good and bad carbs. Refined and processed carbs that have high levels of sugar or bleached (white) flour are bad. On the other hand, complex carbs such as veggies are rich in fiber, low in calories, and leave you feeling satisfied. This includes safe starches such as sweet potatoes, potatoes (russet, red, or gold), yams, and more. Eat smart, make good choices, and be conscious of food combinations so that you are giving your body fuel it can burn.
Cutting calories or eating less frequently helps you to lose weight	In fact, just the opposite is true. Eating more frequently helps to stimulate your body's metabolism and digestion, which burns calories and energy. Not to mention, it keeps you full and satisfied, which means you're less likely to overeat when you do and less likely to experience cravings.
Protein makes you big and bulky	Protein is the building block of muscle tissue. The amino acid profile found in protein is essential. Later in the book, I'll reveal the positive things that come with proper protein consumption. Don't be afraid of protein. Man or woman, it's essential.
Foods labeled "low fat" and "fat free" don't contain calories	As a matter of fact, processed foods with "low fat" or "fat free" labels can contain more calories than the same-size serving of the full-fat version of the product. Don't be fooled by clever marketing or wording in advertisements. Read the labels.
Snacking will make you gain weight	Snacking is not a bad thing. If you're hungry between meals, there's no reason not to snack. Just think about what you are eating. Snacking on sugary, fatty, or high-calorie foods is a bad idea. Period. But healthy snacking, such as eating raw vegetables, lean protein, or nuts and seeds, can fuel your weight loss efforts.
Carb cycling causes muscle loss	Carb cycling, when done correctly, actually preserves and even builds muscle. The Sweet Potato Diet was carefully designed for rapid fat loss, muscle preservation, and lean muscle gains.

You can't eat out and lose weight	Not true. Many restaurants, including "fast food" restaurants, have lower-calorie, healthier menus. There are always alternatives. You just have to be conscious of your food choices when eating out, and make healthier swaps when you need to. i.e.: Grilled chicken for fried or breaded chicken.
You can't eat after a certain time of night and lose weight	Not true (but I can see where this myth started). The problem with eating late at night is in what you choose to eat. Eating high-calorie, sugary foods are not good for your weight loss at any time, but especially not at night when your metabolism has slowed for the day. If you're going to eat later in the evening, eat foods that will help you feel satisfied, but will also stimulate your body to burn calories or build muscle as you recover during sleep.
To be effective, exercise has to take long periods of time	So not true. If you don't have an hour a day to dedicate to exercise (and who does?), you certainly have 10 minutes during the day. You can do effective fat-loss workouts in just 10 minutes (more on that later). If you exercise, even for just a few minutes, you stimulate your body to burn energy for hours after the exercise is done.
Carb cycling doesn't provide enough fiber	Well sure, when done incorrectly, carb cycling doesn't provide enough fiber. This happens when a nutrition plan lacks a sufficient daily amount of veggies or other fibrous foods. This won't be a problem with the Sweet Potato Diet (full of fiber). I even give you a meal planner and a grocery guide.
Carb cycling messes up your metabolism	Oh boy, I love to hate this ridiculous carb cycling myth. Proper carb cycling has the powerful ability to keep your metabolism burning high. It's super effective in preventing fat-loss plateaus. You'll soon see that the Sweet Potato Diet actually allows you to kick-start your sluggish metabolism and burn fat like crazy.

Okay, great. So now we've dismissed those ridiculous myths, it's time to introduce you to the internal furnace: your very own fat-burning machine. Meet your body on the Sweet Potato Diet. But before we do that, I need to address the most critical component to your overall success—mindset.

The Mindset and Awareness for Lasting Success

If losing weight were as simple as just counting calories, we wouldn't have an obesity epidemic on our hands. So what's it all about? You are far more than the sum of your calories. You're a big, biomechanical ball that flourishes when its brain works efficiently and effectively to quiet the mind. Your body always follows what the mind believes and perceives. If you choose success, in any endeavor, you need a mind and body awareness, almost a sixth sense if you will, to question everything and develop the necessary rituals to ensure you succeed.

Life is about finding your grooves and hitting them full swing until they become patterns with little key moments that create new ideas that have the potential to disrupt industries (or your life for now) and change the way people behave. Maybe that isn't fitness for you, but think of your weight loss as a groove and hitting it hard while aware enough to pick out the behaviors that are serving you and continuing to spend as much time each day in that flow as possible. Pretty soon, your health is like getting into your car to go to work in the morning, you don't even think about it, you just do it.

Hmm…like Nike says "Just Do It." It's time, right here to commit to Just Doing It. Who knows, just maybe a new purpose arises from your triumph. That's what happened to me three short years ago after achieving my first goal physique. Now I am on a journey to find the absolute healthiest way of life possible so I can enjoy a beautiful body well into my 100's. I am serious, I choose to live free of medications and oxygen tanks into my 100's. Why not?

Keep something in mind: your bad habits will be lurking, we always tend to go back to what's comfortable to us. It is what it is, but now that you are aware of this, you are as I mention above, equipped to fight them off and replace them with new rituals that will continue to move you towards your goals, in this case fat loss. You'll find that this tool can be used in all areas of your life. As Aristotle said, "The whole is greater than the sum of its parts." When your mind and body are working synergistically, you will feel empowered to take on new challenges. Remember, the only way you can fail is if you give up.

Your Complex Biological Machine

Your amazing body is more complex than any mechanical or high-tech hardware. It constantly uses fuel to power all of its intricate metabolic functions and it needs ongoing maintenance, too. And when you fail to fuel, repair, and maintain your complex machine properly, boy does it show.

You might have noticed some of the signs yourself. Perhaps they are what brought you to this point. Obesity, lack of energy or focus, metabolic dysfunction, or even disease. You see, your body will always do its best to send out warning signs, maybe that's what you're experiencing right now? Stomach pain, chronic fatigue, weight gain, and even diabetes are all warning signs to get your shit together before it's too late!

Don't ignore the first wave of clues, because the second set of warning signs are always more serious and harder to reverse. It's always easier to be proactive than reactive trust me.

So the fact that you're here likely means you're proactive, you're ready to address your health and weight issues, and willing to learn how to naturally work with your body to not only lose fat, but win long-term, too.

Inactivity: Modern Society's Silent Killer

Your body has evolved a little through the ages, but, on the most basic level, it's still very similar to that of your ancestors. You are still compelled by the need to eat in order to survive. This is just fine when you are active, using your body the way it was designed to move and function. But, the trouble is that so many of us still eat even when we are not physically hungry for fuel.

Let's face it, times aren't that tough for most of us. We have plentiful access to food, and the food we get is dense with calories. Hunger is not the issue here. Yet, our "caveman" bodies sometimes revert back to that scarcity mindset, looking for food "just in case" a famine is coming.

While no one expects you to eat like a caveman, we can all learn a lot from their lifestyle. They stayed very active, using their bodies every day and fueled that activity with natural foods from their local environment.

Today, processed foods are all around us, ready to eat in a matter of seconds. Our society has more opportunities to consume calories, yet fewer occasions to burn them off than ever before. We are eating more and doing less.

That's why it's time to change. And I'll show you exactly how to do it.

The Ferris Wheel of Emotional Weight Gain

I'm sure you know what it's like to eat in response to emotion, not hunger. We all do it every day, some more than others. Our modern relationship with food and activity means you really need to master one thing: what drives you to choose the foods you eat?

It's emotion, not hunger, that pushes you to reach for candy. It's habit, not physical needs, that makes you reach for a can of soda.

Master the mental aspect of eating and you will always be one step ahead of "dieting."

Beneath your choices are emotions, not usually very much logic. When you reach for comfort foods because the boss upset you or you feel you deserve a treat; you are not eating to fuel your body. You are using food as self-medication, to pacify your painful emotional problems.

So, let's find new ways to manage your emotions without the mindless eating that causes many of us to spiral out of control.

What can you do to pause, think, and get past that momentary urge to satisfy your emotional hunger? A brisk walk around the block? A tall, cool glass of water? If the emotion you're feeling isn't hunger, no food on earth will satisfy your needs.

Studies show that sugary and fatty foods actually have addictive qualities which will cause you to eat more and more. The end result is weight gain and guilt. And let me tell you, the negative emotions that caused you to overeat don't go away when you eat. They continue to get worse. It's time to take control. It's time to get off this Ferris wheel. Ya feel me?

Movement Is Essential

In order to master your machine, you need to get your mind and body working as one cohesive unstoppable force.

Exercise is a great way to kick-start this synergy and tap into your true potential. Exercise and activity don't just help you lose weight by burning calories. They actually help you manage difficult emotions, cope with stress, and feel more energized.

It's time to start a consistent exercise plan. Exercise does not need to be strenuous to be effective. It should not feel like a chore, and you don't need to "feel the burn" (unless you want to). I don't believe in "no pain, no gain." Remember, we are working with the body here, not against it.

I do believe in "what doesn't challenge you doesn't change you," and with that in mind, I want to encourage you to always challenge yourself throughout this process and throughout life.

Choose an activity you like to do, something you will stick with consistently for the long run. Start with just 3–5 minutes a day (in-place marching first thing in the morning) and you will increase your heart rate and crank up your metabolism. Eventually, you can work up to days where you stay even more active and walk, bike, swim, jog, play a sport, or run around with the kids or the dog for 30 minutes. Remember, it's important to enjoy the journey, if it's not fun you won't stick with it.

Once you start to feel better about your level of fitness, you may even want to join others at your local gym. The accountability you get from working out around others is priceless. At least it was for me. This a great step if you want to take it, but not necessary right out of the gate or ever, if you choose not to.

As your body gets stronger, you may choose to introduce some light resistance training. Training with weights or body weight is extremely beneficial, because you'll continue to burn calories long after your workout, improve bone density, and become less susceptive to injury as you get older.

You do not need to join a gym to do resistance training. You can always pick up a couple of light dumbbells or a set of resistance bands and follow one of my routines on my YouTube channel. PS: My YouTube channel (YouTube.com/morellifit) will be an excellent resource during your journey. I will cover some basic exercises and even give you a few workouts that you can do, with no equipment, right in your living room. Don't worry, they are easy and scalable so that anyone can complete them. Stay tuned—more on that in a few.

Success from Simple Substitutions

A little bit ago, I talked about the old habit of reaching for comfort foods when you're feeling emotional. It's no surprise we call them "comfort" foods. All your mind wants is the relief and satisfaction. This also means that simply cutting out junk foods rarely works. You need to substitute these trick cravings with nourishing foods that satisfy your emotional needs.

It might sound too good to be true, but please trust me: there are lots of healthy alternatives which can provide the same feelings of fullness and contentment without the onslaught of weight gain, bloating, and horrible food hangovers of bingeing on unhealthy foods. It's just a matter of rewiring your brain, and I am going to show you how.

Sugary foods spike your blood sugar levels and give you an instant burst of energy. Unfortunately, your blood sugars then plummet and you experience that horribly familiar "crash." This leads you to eat more sugar in an effort to get high again. It's a cruel cycle most people don't know they are even in, let alone ever get out of.

This cycle sends your body on an addictive roller-coaster ride. The ups are way up, and the downs are way down. What your body really craves is homeostasis, aka balance. A nice, even level without crazy highs or crashing lows.

When we eat foods that help our bodies find natural balance, our intricate machines perform the way they were designed to. There's also another added bonus to eating healthy foods: You can actually eat more often. Lean meat, healthy fats, and complex carbohydrates all take time to digest, so you stay fuller longer and will be much less likely to get hungry, develop cravings, and make poor food choices.

But snacking is important when you do it right. Small meals evenly spaced throughout the day keep your body supplied with a steady stream of healthy nutrients. Many people actually find their cravings for sugar subside naturally after a week or so and they wonder how they ever managed to consume so much of it before.

Keep it Occasional

Does this mean you can never eat any sugary foods again?

It's unrealistic to think that absolutely everyone could go their whole lives without any small sugary treats once in a while. And remember, we are developing a healthy new lifestyle here, not a fad diet you jump onto (then fall off again).

Some people need to indulge occasionally.

If this is you, choose a small, quality sweet and practice portion control. For example, a dark chocolate truffle is much healthier than a bag of Skittles. If you can, choose chocolate with 60% cocoa content (or higher). Keep it under 150 calories and keep it occasional.

If you can't get away from sugar right away, try combining something sweet with something healthy. Dip a banana in chocolate or mix raw nuts with some dark chocolate chips. This provides some nutrients and fiber instead of just empty calories.

Beware calorie-laden soft drinks, fancy coffees, soda, and commercial sports drinks. Even sugar-free sodas are terrible choices for your body. Drink plenty of water with lemon or lime, or caffeine free herbal teas, to hydrate the body and eliminate toxins.

You can do this, I promise. I did it, and I know hundreds of thousands of others who did too.

Start slower if you need to, and wean yourself off the sugars and unhealthy fats. The discomfort is temporary and the rewards are lifelong and amazing, I assure you.

The Surprising Role Integrity Plays in Your Battle Against Fat

Winning at weight loss means making a lot of changes. We've already talked about eating healthier foods, drinking more water, and fitting in more activity. But you know what else it requires? Integrity.

WHAT HAS INTEGRITY GOT TO DO WITH WEIGHT LOSS?

Oprah Winfrey said it best: "Real integrity is doing the right thing, knowing that nobody's going to know whether you did it or not."

Integrity is making a commitment to yourself, regardless of whether anyone else is watching. It involves making a conscious decision to "do the right thing," to no longer cheat yourself by making poor choices while attempting to convince yourself that it doesn't matter.

Why is integrity so powerful in fat-loss success? It forces you to hold yourself accountable. You take control of your life (and your weight), and that provides true and lasting results. You no longer want to engage in behaviors that push you further from your goal. For the first time, you make a real, life-changing commitment to yourself.

This doesn't mean that you're never going to make another bad choice ever again. We are looking for progress, not perfection. But backing your plans with integrity means *you'll take control when you slip.* A tiny lapse doesn't turn into a big binge. Every time you overcome adversity, you get stronger. You're in control now.

INTEGRITY BEGINS WITH NOT MAKING EXCUSES

How many times have you said, "I am going to start tomorrow?" You know tomorrow never comes. Action, today, is what counts. Real life continues, all around challenges present themselves every day, but you remain in control of your choices, which ultimately hold the power to push you towards or pull you away from your goals. It's always your choice.

Maybe you're saying ok, ok Michael, I'll try.

Forget that crap! Stop trying, and start doing. Perhaps Yoda said it best in the movie *Star Wars:* "Do or do not. There is no 'try.'" Your mind doesn't know how to try, it only knows how to do. And if language determines behavior, then what are you saying to yourself?

Saying "I'll try" is giving yourself a way out. Today, you start choosing your destiny. Trying is gone, eliminate it from your vocabulary along with "ifs," "buts," and "coulda" "woulda" and "shoulda." These words will never serve you. You're not a victim anymore. You haven't been defeated. You have a new blueprint that works and you will win if you choose to, period!

Remember the promises you made to yourself when you bought this book.

The New You One Commitment at a Time

A failsafe approach is to look at the commitment you've made to yourself by honoring just one small promise at a time. You're less likely to feel overwhelmed or anxious. You'll steadily work your way through the obstacles, becoming strong and fearless in your pursuit. As the bond between you and your integrity strengthens, your mind and body become one, and something magical happens. You start checking off one box after another.

Move over! Now you've got some serious momentum, you're riding your groove, you're productive, you're seeing progress, and most importantly you're in control.

Did you know that the world's top athletes, like gold medal and likely the most prolific Olympian in history Michael Phelps, understand that visualization is key to winning? Google him and check out his visualization rituals, no wonder he's the most decorated Olympian in history.

Just like Michael Phelps and all of the other uber-successful people in this world, it's important to begin with the end in mind. Can you see yourself crossing the finish line (goal number one) of your new journey? What does it look like? Who are you with? Where are you at? Are there any smells? Are you tasting anything?

I know this sounds crazy, but the more intense the visualization, the more likely you are to achieve success—this goes for anything you choose to go after in life.

Take five minutes to do this exercise with me now.

Imagine yourself at your goal weight. Your health has improved and you can run without shortness of breath. If you have kids, now you're keeping up with them on a daily basis.

How do you feel when you get up in the morning? How do you feel when you go to bed after a healthy, active day? What's it feel like to have your old clothes finally fit again? What do your relationships look like? What are your family and friends saying?

Do not proceed until you've visualized your goals.

Ok then. Now that you know exactly (down to the smell) where you are going, you can finally get there. It's time to start living it.

It's all in the simple, daily disciplines. Remember, they are easy to do, but just as easy not to do. You've seen your future. Think about it often, and be patient and consistent enough to break the tape at your finish line.

SMART and Easy Ways That Help You Knock Out Fat

Combine the above with this little set of behaviors and solidify your success.

Build these in as daily habits (one at a time, of course), and increase the likelihood of success in your life tenfold.

SET "SMARTER" GOALS

Goal-setting is vital, as I just mentioned, and the visualization part is key. The Sweet Potato Diet is designed to help you burn fat every month. But you have to follow it.

Alongside the goals I've set inside this program, you should have your own goals to review as the weeks progress. Setting personal goals will keep you motivated, give you direction, and help you make the right decisions when temptation knocks. Your goals are the road map to your fat-loss, and a healthy lifestyle in your new body is the destination.

FIVE-STEP STRATEGY FOR SHORT- AND LONG-TERM GOALS

Here's exactly how I set personal goals. It's worked for me, so give it a go.

1. Write down your goals, and be really specific. One study, led by Dr. Gail Matthews, a psychology professor at Dominican University in California, concluded that people who wrote down their goals and made themselves accountable to someone else were on average 33% more successful in accomplishing their target than those who just set goals.

2. List the three most important steps that you'll need to take to realize your goal. Number them by order of importance.

3. Set specific dates for each goal. Turn the dates into mini milestones with small rewards for each. For example, *"It's January 21st, 30 days from today,*

and I have lost 11 pounds and 2 inches off my waist." A goal without a deadline is merely a wish. Don't fool yourself.

4. Take action right away to avoid the "shoulda, woulda, couldas". Get going now. As momentum builds, you'll see results, and results foster a sense of control, which leads to progress.

5. Make a daily checklist. Include all of the simple, daily disciplines you can do consistently.

There are no shortcuts to fat loss and fitness. Prepare, commit, and win.

BANISH NEGATIVE STRESS

Setting goals naturally brings on a little of the "good" stress into your life, as you strive to make changes for the better. Focus on your simple, daily disciplines today. Don't worry about tomorrow or next week. Nothing ever happened in the past, or will happen in the future, that didn't first happen in the now. The "now" is all you really ever have.

There's a saying that I love: "Don't let tomorrow's worry overshadow today's accomplishments."

Here's a great question I read, and that is the premise behind Gary Keller's book *The One Thing,* and I find myself asking it every day when I wake up.

What's the one thing I can do, such that by doing it, it makes everything else easier or unnecessary? Ask the question and add in whatever your focus is for the day, for example "makes my fat loss easier."

Today is your only focus—period.

Stress, or what we have labeled anxiety, often sneaks in when we focus on the future or our unrealistic expectations. When you find yourself out in lala land, bring your focus back to the present. You casted your vision, you saw it, now the only way you can get there is through the now.

BE PATIENT

Patience is extremely important when it comes to achieving success.

Avoid trying to accelerate your fat loss. Super-fast, short-term results are usually followed by long-term disappointment. Remember: the habits, strategies, and disciplines provided in the Sweet Potato Diet are there to help you create a sustainable lifestyle that will not only help you lose fat, but keep it off…for life.

Be patient; you never know how close you are to your next breakthrough.

BE THOROUGH AND USE MY RESOURCES

It's a good idea to re-read all the material in *The Sweet Potato Diet*. Let it sink in. Eat it (pun intended, haha!), breathe it, live it, and make sure to visit SweetPotatoDiet.com for additional support and new resources.

KEEP PHOTOGRAPHIC RECORDS

When you are in the midst of a body transformation, two things are certain: you will have good days and bad days, and you may at times struggle to recognize just how far you've come. I know, because I've been there. Not only are we our worst critics, but we see ourselves every day, so it's hard for us to notice change.

Taking photos at regular intervals will help. The pictures will document your progress, and there's no motivation like going back and looking at pictures from when you first started and seeing the body composition changes.

Here are my best tips for taking great photos:

1. Use a digital or high-quality phone camera. Sharp, clear pictures are the best way to provide clear, indisputable evidence (to yourself or others) of your physical transformation.

2. Take the pictures in a well-lit area against a solid background. This will create clear images where your body's subtle changes can be easily distinguished as the series of photos progress.

3. Wear the same or similar clothing. You should wear the type of clothing that either reveals your body or makes your body's lines and characteristics easily distinguishable. This will make it easier to spot changes in your physique.

5. Take photos from various angles. Taking your photos from a combination of angles will reveal your face shape and the outlines of your body. I recommend a front view, back view, and a side view. This will give you a comprehensive outlook as you progress on your journey.

6. Take pictures at regular intervals. I advise monthly pictures as an invaluable way to see the physical changes. When you compare your photos side-by-side, the images will reveal some very exciting body composition changes.

TRACK YOUR PROGRESS

It's been said that "you can only improve what you measure."

This is the principle of success in small steps that I used throughout my own transformation.

Tracking your progress is a powerful tool: it keeps you focused on your goals, allows you to see any slight deviations, and helps you make corrections much quicker.

You'll also find that tracking progress helps to minimize stress, encouraging you to be patient as you move closer and closer to your goals. You can see them, right? I sure can!

I also suggest recording your meals (at least for the first month). It doesn't take very long, and later in *The Sweet Potato Diet,* I'll show you exactly how. Don't worry, it's super simple.

Look back every two weeks, analyze your information and your results. In other words, take a quick audit. Then, based on your findings, you will know exactly what little tweaks can be made to be even more efficient on your journey.

Sweet Potato Diet Example Food Log

NOTE: Put down everything you eat in a current day, be honest, and don't forget your snacks! You want a real picture of what you're working with.

BREAKFAST	Bagel with low fat cream cheese Starbucks Frappuccino
MORNING SNACK	1 string cheese stick and 1 Strawberry Nutri-Grain bar
LUNCH	Subway 6' Chicken Teriyaki Sub Bag of Lays potato chips Diet Coke
AFTERNOON SNACK	Yoplait Lite yogurt
DINNER	Spaghetti and grilled shrimp Side of green beans Glass of milk
NIGHTTIME SNACK	7 Chips Ahoy! cookies
WATER	○ ○ ○ ○ ○ ○ ○ ○ ○ ○ ○ ○ ○ ○

Food Log / Meal Planner

	MONDAY	TUESDAY	WEDNESDA
BREAKFAST			
MORNING SNACK			
LUNCH			
AFTERNOON SNACK			
DINNER			
NIGHTTIME SNACK			
WATER	○○○○○ ○○○○○ ○○○○○	○○○○○ ○○○○○ ○○○○○	○○○○○ ○○○○○ ○○○○○

THURSDAY	FRIDAY	SATURDAY	SUNDAY
○○○○○ ○○○○○ ○○○○○	○○○○○ ○○○○○ ○○○○○	○○○○○ ○○○○○ ○○○○○	○○○○○ ○○○○○ ○○○○○

Victory Is Yours... Only When You Prepare for It

If you were planning a road trip, you would have a map (or GPS) up front and a spare tire in the trunk. I think we can all agree that without these basic preparations, your chances of failure increase substantially. It's simple logic, if you don't know where you are going, you could end up anywhere.

The same applies to your fat-loss goals. Lack of preparation can turn the simplest tasks into a lengthy and extended journey. Have you ever taken a trip that should have been just 10 minutes and yet, without directions turned out to be three times that long? This leads to frustration and it can easily get out of hand and end in failure.

Perhaps your previous efforts at weight loss haven't involved proper planning. You've heard the saying "fail to prepare, and prepare to fail." This couldn't be more true. In fact, almost always it's a lack of preparation. That's all about to change as we set some solid groundwork for your journey on the Sweet Potato Diet.

Simply deciding that you are going to change your diet isn't enough—as we have talked about, you need to take small steps to ensure your success. Everything you've read so far has laid the emotional and psychological foundations for your success. Now, it's time for some quick fit fundamentals to reinforce your new lifestyle.

Here are my favorite practical preparation strategies for victory.

ELIMINATE THE GARBAGE

If you've looked at the grocery lists, you know by now exactly what foods to stock up on. It's also critical to eliminate the wrong ones. If you have sugary or fatty foods in your house, you will at some point likely eat them—they're addictive, remember?

Hit all your secret stashes, too. You need to purge your desk drawer, gym bag, and the console of your car. Get rid of it all! Next, take the time to prepare and replace that junk with healthy snacks. You can use reusable containers to take with you on-the-go. I like julienned carrots, celery with almond butter, hard boiled eggs, sweet potato halves, or a handful of nuts when I need a snack. Turkey or grass-fed beef jerky are also some of my favorite on-the-go snacks.

Here are the foods you definitely want to ditch before you start your weight-loss journey. Remember, what you don't have around, you can't eat.

- Alcohol
- Bakery products—especially white bread
- Bottled/canned sauces and salad dressings
- Candy
- Cereal bars
- Chips
- Cookies
- Crackers
- Dried fruit
- Fried foods
- Fruit juice
- Ice cream
- Pre-prepped frozen meals—even if labeled "diet" or "healthy"
- Soda—it's proven to cause health problems due to sugar levels and sugar substitutes

Also, ditch all foods with the following ingredients on the label:

- High fructose corn syrup (HFCS)
- Hydrogenated oils or shortening
- White flour
- White sugar

It's critical that you buy and stock up on the right foods for your journey. You are what you eat. If you choose results, you must give your body the foods required to boost your metabolism and allow it to run well.

It is time to start looking at food in a new way. Think of your purchases as buying the best fuel for your trip. Fuel that burns slowly and steadily is preferable to that which gives you a short blast of energy. Highly-efficient and slow-burning foods are proteins, veggies, some nuts, and certain fruits. Use the Approved Foods List and Grocery Guide at the end of the book to help you stock your home, your office, and your car.

Keep in mind, sugars are very inefficient forms of fuel. They blast you with a quick burst of energy and then leave you wanting more. A study published by the American Diabetes Association links sugar, particularly in drinks, with spikes in our blood sugar which lead to metabolic syndrome and type 2 diabetes.

Processed foods are full of sugar to make a product more appealing. In the September 2013 issue of the *American Journal of Clinical Nutrition*, a study stated that the brain patterns of people eating high fat and sugar foods are similar to those that occur in people who take heroin and cocaine. Crazy, right?

Sugars and fats are also hidden in the foods we eat. Don't be fooled by claims that a food is healthy or natural. These packaged foods can still be high in unhealthy ingredients.

Stock up on lean meats, nuts and seeds, safe starches like sweet potatoes (of course!), a little bit of fruit, and tons of vegetables. Frozen fruits and vegetables are another option as long as there are no added ingredients or sugars. Avoid the heavily-processed packages. A good rule of thumb that works in most cases is the more ingredients something has, the less likely it is to be healthy. Look for things that you cannot pronounce, Google them, and make the smart choice.

We are all tempted to eat the wrong things at times. You need to plan ahead with coping strategies, including something you can do as a substitute or replacement. Visualization is a powerful technique. Play back these scenarios in your head over and over again so when the time comes that you are tempted, you know how to handle it.

The April 2014 *NIH Record* summarized ground-breaking work by Dr. Leonard H. Epstein of the University at Buffalo. Epstein says addiction to sweets is as much to do with the brain as it is to do with physical cravings.

When you eat sugary foods, the brain's reward system focuses on the perceived value of these foods, so you want to eat them more often. To break this pattern, Epstein suggests shifting your focus towards a positive event, so you can train your brain to steer away from its fixation with unhealthy foods. Epstein states that the results depend on how vividly you can imagine the positive effects of the event.

RECRUIT YOUR TRIBE

When you are embarking on your weight loss journey, it's important to prepare the others that will be traveling with you.

Before you start, let your loved ones know what you are doing and how they can be supportive during your journey. This can be as simple as asking them not to bring junk food into the house or eat late at night when you are trying not to.

Research shows that your social group is one of the most important factors in your success. *The New England Journal of Medicine* found that obesity is influenced by the people closest to you. Your chances of becoming obese increase by 57% if you have a friend who is obese and by 37% if your spouse is obese.

While you would love everyone to be on board with your weight-loss journey, sometimes other people aren't interested. So, what do you do if someone you need support from is not all that crazy about helping you?

COMMUNICATE WITH THOSE CLOSEST TO YOU

Communication with the person closest to you in life is vital. Some partners may resent your weight-loss plan as it puts their health and weight under scrutiny, too. Changes in your life can force others to think about their current state. Our changes can potentially bring attention to changes they need to make themselves. Change is hard for a lot of people, and just because you are ready to change doesn't mean they are. And sometimes that can cause others to feel resentful.

But someone who loves you will want the best for you. Clinical studies confirm that carrying extra weight can lead to health issues such as coronary heart disease, type 2 diabetes, cancer, high blood pressure, and even stroke. Loved ones don't want you to face that. When someone who might be resentful at first decides to open up, the best thing you can do is lead them to the information you received before making your change. That way they can understand not only the place you started in, but the destination you want to reach.

Have an open, honest discussion with them about your fears and goals. They will see that your desire to lose weight goes deeper than trying to look different. Being healthier and feeling better are good motivators. Who knows, they may even be inspired by your determination.

Neutralizing Your Triggers

We all have triggers that set us off on and down a destructive path. Whether it is stress or emotion, these likely have become habits over time. We all have the urge to reach for the wrong foods at times.

All triggers work the same. The trigger is the cue to the action or behavior which ultimately leads to some reward at the end (rewards aren't always good, even though our intentions may be). For example, if you binge at night, you must identify the trigger that cued the behavior that you choose to end. Stress, boredom, or if you're like me and have kids, them misbehaving could even be your trigger. It's stress, right? You cope with it by opening up the cabinets.

Once you recognize the trigger that causes this action, then you can more easily identify it and adjust your routine for better results. For example, when the trigger occurs, go outside for a quick walk, or go and pet your dog. Seriously. Replace the behavior with the new behavior and after several times you'll be doing the new more productive behavior in favor of the old. The idea is that eventually, you start subconsciously doing your new behavior without thinking about it and then it becomes a positive routine.

Take the time to think about when your food triggers occur and what you can do to combat them. Here are some common triggers to consider:

TRIGGER: FOOD

If having a coffee makes you want to eat a croissant, find a new beverage for now. If eating a baked potato means you have to slather on sour cream, eat something else instead. The trick lies in switching up your habits. Reduce your portions. And treat yourself by enjoying the "reward meals" built into the Sweet Potato Diet.

TRIGGER: IRRITATING PEOPLE

Some people just get under your skin. Recognize this, acknowledge it, because pushing it down will not help. Instead, remember that you do not identify with what people say about you. You are so much more than that. And if you find yourself struggling emotionally to let go of something negative someone else said, find someone who does support you and ask for positive reinforcement. Just talking to someone positive can be enough to make you feel better.

TRIGGER: BOREDOM

When we are sitting around doing nothing, we are more likely to eat. Get up and go for a walk, clean up the dinner dishes, or tidy up some papers. Busy hands can't grab for food. Chew on a stick of gum or brush your teeth to discourage eating. Also, drinking a cup of water can help.

TRIGGER: DINING OUT

Dining out and allowing yourself a treat is okay sometimes. But, this has to be occasional, not a habit. Consider dining out only for your reward meals. And remember, there are always healthier choices on the menu like a salad, a steak dinner with veggies, or a stir fry. Avoid bread, and if you want to have a dessert, try splitting it with someone to slash your calories. In Phase 1, we encourage you to avoid eating out until you establish good habits and routines. In Phase 2, we encourage you to only eat out on cheat meals and to use the knowledge you have gained in Phase 1 to make the best choices. Read the section "Food on the Go" for ideas about dining out or any other worst-diet-case scenarios where you are not prepared with food.

TRIGGER: SOCIAL EVENTS

Those little sausages and snacks at a party can add up quickly. If you know there will be food at a social event, eat something healthy before you go, drink plenty of water, and grab a low-cal drink when you get there. Or, instead of drinking alcohol, order a sparkling water on the rocks and toss in a lemon and lime. This can look like a drink, save you the calories, give your liver a break, and let you enjoy the party.

TRIGGER: THE OFFICE

Office vending machines and the daily run to the local coffee shop can be tempting if you don't prepare ahead of time. Take your healthy snacks to the office and drink a lot of water. Water not only hydrates, but helps manage your appetite, too.

Losing weight is about changing habits. These steps will help you lose weight and keep it off for good.

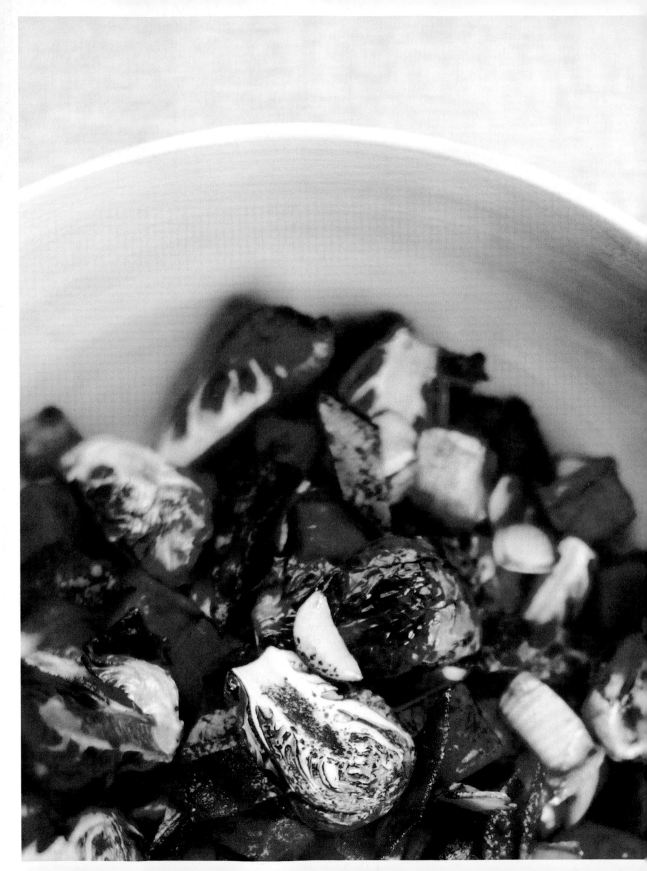

CHAPTER 2:

Core Eating Principles

I n this section on Core Eating and Nutrition Principles, you'll find everything you need in order to increase fat loss and overall health, including information on proteins, carbs, and fats and the important role they all play in the Sweet Potato Diet.

Consider this your bible for nutrition. This is an incredible resource that I only wish I had when I first started, and it will set you up for major success. So, be sure to take the time to review and implement everything before moving on. Trust me on this, don't skip through this part.

What to Eat?

The Sweet Potato Diet's nutrition principles are built on a solid foundation of macro- and micro-nutrients. Each one plays a critical role in your health and well-being. And that's crucial to your success with this program.

MACRONUTRIENTS VERSUS MICRONUTRIENTS

Macronutrients are the energy-containing nutrients: proteins, fats, and carbohydrates. Micro-nutrients are all the vitamins and minerals within foods. They're responsible for organ function, cell growth, food utilization, and so much more.

PROTEINS, FATS, AND CARBS

Of the three macronutrients, carbohydrates are the only ones that are not essential. That means you could live a perfectly healthy life if you never ate another carbohydrate again. However, I don't suggest doing that because carbohydrates are an excellent source of fuel when intake is properly managed, as we teach you to do on the Sweet Potato Diet.

Proteins and fats are essential. As you'll see below, they play a vital role in everything from increasing metabolism to regulating hormones.

Eating Frequency

Eating meals and snacks consistently throughout the day is going to be important to your fat-loss success. But the right snacks. When we hear the word "snack," we think chips and bars—no.

My preferred meal frequency—and the one I tend to recommend to clients—is five small meals. That's what I'd like you to try as you get used to the Sweet Potato Diet way of eating. Five meals per day gives you consistency without huge gaps between meals. You shouldn't get hungry, and your body will enjoy a steady stream of nutrients.

FAT BURNING WAYS TO SNACK

Snacking is not a bad thing on the Sweet Potato Diet (I bet you're glad to hear that). In fact, snacking is a great way to keep your meal frequency consistent and avoid the onset of cravings.

Fat and protein combinations are especially filling at snack times. I know I briefly mentioned them previously, but these are some of my favorite go-to snack ideas:

1. Quality beef jerky
2. Hard boiled eggs
3. Veggie sticks
4. Tuna and veggies
5. Almond butter and apple
6. Nut mixes (be sure to practice portion control)
7. Chicken breast
8. Cubed sweet potato with spices

9. Canned pumpkin, vanilla protein powder, sliced almonds, chia seeds, and cinnamon (this is lower fat but stays pretty low-carb too, thanks to the pumpkin)

Switch It Up: Why Variety Is Important

Want to know what I've noticed? Once people start eating clean, they tend to fall into the trap of eating the same foods all the time. While this is certainly better than going back to the junk, variety is important.

Here's why.

Lack of variety presents a couple of problems.

#1 INSUFFICIENT NUTRIENTS, VITAMINS, AND MINERALS

A diet that lacks variety is also going to lack the complete spectrum of micronutrients, vitamins, and minerals available to us if we eat a full range of natural, whole foods.

#2 POTENTIAL FOOD INTOLERANCES

The second problem is the potential development of food intolerances, specifically to wheat proteins. The potential varies from person to person, but if you are exposed to allergens every day, you can develop intolerances.

SOMETIMES SEEING YOUR OPTIONS IS ALL IT TAKES

For some people, it can be hard to come up with different ideas, especially for breakfast.

But one great way to change things up is to write down several options for your proteins, carbohydrates, and fats for each meal. Try to write down at least 3–5 different options for each, and then as you go through the week, you can check off foods you have eaten a few times and see what other options you might have missed.

Reference the Approved Foods List and Grocery Guide to get ideas of foods that you might not have even thought of. This little guide is gold!

TRY SOMETHING UNUSUAL

Start buying foods you normally wouldn't think of trying. In fact, if you see something and you have no idea what the heck it's used for, or where it's grown for that matter, buy it, take it home, and Google a recipe for it. You'll be surprised at what you find. You may have to get a bit adventurous with your shopping. Live a little, would ya?

The Importance Of Water Intake for Fat Loss

Healthy drinking is easy, right? As long as you're chugging plenty of water, it's all good. Well, not quite. Hydration for fat loss is often overlooked, so let's make sure you know how much to drink on a daily basis.

Even if it seems as though your hydration status is solid, I advise you to keep track of it so you can really get it dialed in. I often think I am drinking more than I actually am. Keeping track shows me exactly how I'm doing.

A SIMPLE HYDRATION FORMULA

The formula I use for optimal hydration:

½ the number of pounds of body weight (BW) in ounces per day (1 ounce = 29.5mL) (So, 200 lbs = 100 oz)

This way you'll replace fluid lost throughout the day due to normal sweat and increased metabolism and keep your body's natural fat-loss ability ticking over. Proper hydration clears the metabolic waste from your system and keeps your digestion running right.

When the body is chronically dehydrated, it holds on to water for survival. The body is very efficient at retaining water. No one wants to be holding water, so constantly hydrate. This will ensure that your body doesn't hang on to excess water. This will make you feel better, enhance muscle tone, and work in your favor to show off your efforts on the Sweet Potato Diet. Ever since I have increased my water intake, I get less headaches, less hunger cravings, and I appear leaner because my body doesn't hang on to as much water. Don't overlook daily water intake.

NOTE: *Drinks like iced tea and diet sodas DO NOT count toward your hydration for the day. On the approved foods list, you will see other liquids that I have approved, however, they DO NOT count towards your daily water intake—they are a bonus.*

HYDRATION TIMING AND STRATEGY

The timing of your hydration is important. Large amounts of water during meals can dilute gastric acids and enzymes, leading to inefficient digestion. Try not to drink anything during meals or for 30 minutes after eating to optimize digestion. Remember, all you can do is your best. When you're properly hydrated this becomes much easier.

Relax, chew your food, and let your saliva break it down. Sure, there are times when liquid is needed to help food go down, so sip a little. But don't chug water during meals. All the healthy eating in the world will do you little good if the food is poorly digested.

You can even give this a go. Drink 8 ounces of water 20 to 30 minutes before your meal to increase saliva content and help digestion.

COFFEE—FRIEND OR FOE?

It's okay to have a little coffee in your diet. I love a really good espresso. Despite being demonized as a diuretic, it's no bad thing. Coffee is a known ergogenic (training aid) that contains a fair amount of antioxidants, as well as caffeine. Caffeine is actually a fantastic all-natural fat burner which can really help your fat loss efforts. It's the very reason I created my own line, MorellisCoffee.com coffee and drink it every morning. I often consume it about 30 minutes before my workouts.

Too many people take energy pills containing harmful chemicals when all they need is a shot of espresso or a cup of black coffee. The main downfall of our hefty coffee consumption is all the extra stuff people add to it (sugar, creamer, sprinkles, milk, and syrups). Actual coffee itself is not the bad guy. Choose organic beans, always. Coffee is the most heavily-sprayed crop on the planet, you do not want to ingest all of those pesticides.

That said, coffee does cause gastric motility, which can be unpleasant or downright troublesome for anyone with a delicate gut. If over-consumed, it can also cause problems with your adrenals, so consume moderately. Tea is an even better option.

BENEFITS OF ALL TYPES OF TEA

These days, we have loads of different types of tea to choose from, including green, white, and rooibos, as well as traditional black tea. Green tea is another fantastic natural thermogenic (fat burner). This is thanks to its naturally high levels of catechins, natural compounds which function as antioxidants and thermogenics, and its levels of theanine, a precursor to a calming neurotransmitter.

Rooibos tea is actually an African bush that comes in green and red. It contains no caffeine, but is very high in antioxidants. Black teas and herbal teas are fine to drink when you're living the Sweet Potato Diet fat-loss lifestyle, too. You should see my tea collection at home; we've got dozens of herbal, green, and Rooibos teas, and the whole family enjoys them all. Who needs soda?

AVOID THE ALCOHOL PITFALL

Alcohol consumption can really slam the brakes on your fat loss for a number of reasons. It has a negative effect on hydration, contains empty calories (7 calories per gram of alcohol), is packed with sugar, and often leads to cravings for unhealthy foods. It also affects fatty acid synthesis, testosterone production (both men and women want to keep that high for fat loss), and can impact your sleep, too.

All of the above are essential for health, fat loss, and better body composition. But we are social creatures. I just want you to be aware of alcohol's damaging effects and consider cutting it out (or at least cutting back) now that you've made the commitment to a healthier way of life.

If you choose to drink while on this program, then don't consume more than 1 to 2 drinks per week and make smart choices like clear spirits or organic wines. When I drink, I keep it to one, two glasses max, and always buy my wine from the same place—DryFarmWines.com /morellifit.

The benefits of red wine for general health have been studied to an extensive degree despite being quite minimal. Red wine does include antioxidants, and can be enjoyed in moderation.

I like to look at my nutrition this way: whatever I choose to consume will either be used for fuel or repair. Will this food or drink help or hinder me? Alcohol negatively affects hormonal response and that's usually all I need to think about in order to keep it to a minimum.

Sweeteners: The Natural Alternative to Sugar

Refined sugar (table sugar) is not good for you or your weight-loss goals.

If you needed refined table sugar to pay you in nutrients, it couldn't. It's flat broke. Sugar is a tough one to completely eliminate from your diet, believe me I know. At the very least, swap it for some better alternatives. There are some really good all-natural sweeteners starting with Stevia.

STEVIA

Stevia is a low-calorie sweetener derived from the leaves of the *Stevia rebaudiana* plant found in South America. In studies, Stevia has actually been shown to have health benefits, including lowering blood sugar levels in diabetics. Stevia is the one we use most at our house, we get the liquid drops and use them quite frequently.

XYLITOL

Xylitol is a sugar alcohol that has approximately two-thirds the calories contained in sugar and is similar to sugar in sweetness. Xylitol does not raise insulin or blood sugar levels.

UNREFINED COCONUT SUGAR

Unrefined coconut sugar is also a good alternative because it has not gone through all of the processing that table sugar has and hasn't been stripped of its nutritional value. Unrefined coconut sugar is also low on the glycemic index and does not spike your blood sugar when used in moderation. Coconut sugar is excellent for baking.

THE TRUTH ABOUT MILK

Milk is only essential for two types of people:

1. People trying to gain weight
2. People who want to get sick

I learned this during my education at OPEX fitness. And that statement usually throws people off. But hear me out. (You know I don't get my kicks from upsetting people.)

It's a valid statement.

Milk is highly anabolic and causes a large insulin release, hence its long-term possible outcome having carcinogenic properties. Lactose—the protein found in milk—isn't terrible (although it often causes inflammatory issues), but it can be problematic for some people, even if they aren't lactose intolerant.

For example, I am not lactose intolerant, but milk does give me some problems. After drinking milk a few times I find my sinuses full of mucus and sometimes have a "phlegmy" feeling. This is a great reason to cut out certain foods that might be problematic for you, for at least just a few weeks. When you reintroduce them, you are more likely to notice how they affect your body and can then make the best decisions for your body. You won't find much dairy on our lists.

With that in mind, is there any point in drinking milk?

The "calcium" argument for milk is highly overstated when you consider North Americans consume some of the highest levels of milk in the world, yet have the highest rates of osteoporosis.

David S. Ludwig, MD, PhD, published an article on milk and calcium in the September 2013 edition of *JAMA Pediatrics*. Dr. Ludwig points out there are many other calcium sources than milk, and countries that don't consume milk actually have a lower rate of bone fractures.

And it probably won't surprise you by now to hear that the quality of grocery store milk is quite low, due in large part to high-heat pasteurization, homogenization, and the way dairy cattle are fed, farmed, and raised. I consume dairy in extreme moderation and I suggest, you at the very least, consider removing it for a few weeks to see the difference, from there you can gauge your consumption.

The Secret Weapon for Successful Weight Loss (It's Not What You Think)

What's the one single thing that makes for successful weight loss?

Is it calorie counting? No.

Cutting out a food group? No.

EATING LESS OFTEN? DEFINITELY NOT

It's a simple habit everyone can start working on right now: portion size. One of the most important components of successfully losing weight—and keeping it off for life—is to regulate and be mindful of the sizes of your meals.

PORTION SIZE 20 YEARS AGO		
Regular sized soda drink:	6.5 ounces	85 calories
Box of popcorn:	5 cups	270 calories
A large pizza:	Two slices	500 calories
Bagel:	3 inches	140 calories
Muffin:	1.5 ounces	210 calories
Chicken Caesar salad:	1 ½ cups	390 calories
Cheesecake:	3 ounces	260 calories

PORTION SIZE TODAY		
Regular sized soda drink:	20 ounces	250 calories
Popcorn Tub:	11 cups	630 calories
A large pizza:	Two slices	850 calories
Bagel:	6 inches	350 calories
Muffin:	4 ounces	500 calories
Chicken Caesar salad:	3 ½ cups	790 calories
Cheesecake:	7 ounces	640 calories

(*Source: National Institutes of Health; National Heart, Lung and Blood Institute. Parent **TIPS:** Portion Size Matters; Portion Distortion Quiz)

Did you know that the meal portions we are served today in restaurants are often twice the size they were 20 years ago*? Check out these scary stats:

WOW. What a difference 20 years makes. But of course, our bodies, DNA, and hormones haven't changed in 20 years. In fact, our activity levels have actually gone down with an increase of television time and the use of devices. It's no wonder our bodies can't keep up with the onslaught of calories.

We have become accustomed to very large portion sizes without really thinking about how it affects our ability to maintain a normal and healthy body weight. As you begin to lose weight, you need to be mindful of this. It can make or break your goals.

MEASURING YOUR PORTIONS

As you begin shedding body fat during the Sweet Potato Diet, we will be asking you (in Phase 2 only) to use your hands to measure your portion sizes. This will ensure that you are choosing the correct portions. See, we kept it super simple, no calorie counting, and no food scales or measuring cups. This will help not only at home, but also on the go, at restaurants, and at cafes when you are out and about.

And, because your hands are proportionate to your body, it's the perfect way to ensure you are eating exactly the right amount at all times.

LEARNING TO USE YOUR HANDS

Learn how to calculate portion sizes using your hands. Here's what we suggest in order to get the very best results from the Sweet Potato Diet.

- Proteins (meat or poultry): Recommended serving size is 3 ounces. This is equal to the size of the palm of your hand.
- Carbohydrates: Recommended serving size is 1 cup. This is equal to the size of your clenched fist.
- Vegetables: Recommended serving size is approximately 2 cups of vegetables. This is equal to the size of two clenched fists.
- Fats: Recommended serving size is 1 tablespoon. This is equal to the tip of your thumb, approximately from the joint to the tip.
- Flavorings (spices and seasonings): Use these to your liking on your meals.

ANATOMY *of a* SERVING

ALL MEASUREMENTS ARE EQUVALENT TO 1 SERVING

FATS
FULL THUMB
2 TABLESPOONS

PROTEIN
FULL PALM
3 OUNCES

CARBS / VEGETABLES
FISTED HAND (1 FOR CARBS, 2 FOR VEGETABLES)
1 CUP

Food Preparation: Your Simple 3-Step System for Success

Do you want to know why I think most people fail at diets, despite their best intentions? Failure to plan and prepare. Food preparation is key. I'm going to let you in on my very best secrets. Setting aside the time all at once saves time throughout the week and allows you to stay on track. These food prep secrets have been a life saver to so many clients, if it weren't for these, many would have failed.

It's so dang easy to stop and grab something quick when you're on the go and don't have anything handy. Don't let yourself get to that stage.

Here's what I suggest:

Choose one day a week as food-prep day. I suggest making Sundays the day, but use whatever day works best for you.

1. Cook a boatload of meat and put it in ziploc bags. You could grab a large pack of chicken breasts from your favorite grocery store. Toss them on a George Foreman grill with a bit of lemon and black pepper, and you'll have delicious, quality protein ready for the entire week. Also, by preportioning your meals into Tupperware, you can get all of your meats, carbs, and veggies into containers that are complete meals-to-go.

2. Use a similar approach for your veggies. Chop up a bunch of different veggies (carrots, celery, red pepper, or cucumbers) and place them into Tupperware containers or toss them into some ziploc bags. Do the same for your to-go snacks. Separately bag portions of blueberries, hard boiled eggs, and nuts for an easy-to-reach-for snack. They will be ready to go when you are.

3. At the start of each day, just grab and go. When you get hungry, you'll have nutrient-dense, low-calorie foods handy. Boom. It's that easy.

Food on-the-Go

Now that you have food-prep handled, remember to take it with you. Preparing food ahead of time helps you fight through temptation and cravings.

If you're "on-the-go," having your prepared food with you eliminates the temptation to grab foods that aren't a part of your regular meal plan. Whether you're out at work, going to class, or running errands, the vending machine, coffee shop, and corner store won't need your cash.

If you get a food craving or feel super hungry, the on-the-go-plan food is right there. Again, you won't need to eat anything that's not part of the plan.

Here are some examples of prepared foods for my on-the-go days:

- baked chicken
- chicken breast slices
- turkey
- sliced roast beef
- beef jerky
- hard boiled eggs
- canned fish or chicken
- grass-fed protein shakes
- raw vegetables or veggie sticks
- homemade protein balls
- raw nuts or nut mixes
  (no sugar added)

Please take your coach's advice (that's me, by the way) and get into the great habit of prepping meals, snacks, and on-the-go food every week. It has been one of the biggest factors for all of my clients staying successful on the Sweet Potato Diet.

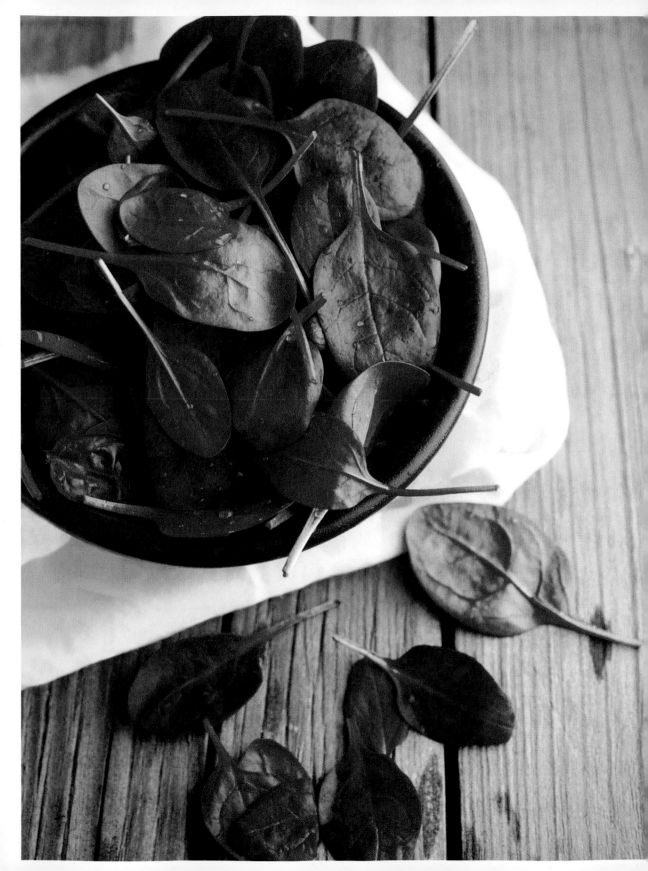

CHAPTER 3:

Understanding Super Carbs and Essential Nutrition

Super Carbs: Fruits, Greens, Roots, and Tubers

VEGETABLES

There is no limit to the amount of vegetables that we can eat on this plan, because cruciferous veggies do not affect the glycemic index. Typically, it takes more energy to break down these vegetables than they give your body. These are considered "non-active" or free carbs. They also do not affect blood sugar levels.

There are other huge upsides to eating large amounts of vegetables on a diet. Vegetables are nutrient dense and have a lot of volume so you not only feel fuller when you eat them, you stay fuller for longer. Veggies fill you up without extra calories and this make them great for snacking and holding you over until your next meal. This is why you get two fists full at every meal. In the event you get hungry, feel free to eat as many as you'd like.

FRUITS

Fruits are not to be eaten as vegetables, because even though they are nutritious, fruits have fructose, which is a form of sugar. And while it's natural, sugar is still sugar, and the consequences are important ones to consider, especially when you are choosing to lose fat.

I remember when I first got started three years ago, I would ask my clients to send in their 3–5 day food logs so I could see where their troubles were. Ninety-five percent of the time those that couldn't lose fat or that were stuck were always eating way too many servings of fruit.

Are fruits all bad? No. They are nutrient dense and packed with antioxidants. They are good for your overall health and a good source of healthy energy. And they are always my recommended go-to when you have a sweet-tooth craving you need to knock out. I mean, it's always better to grab an apple instead of a Snickers bar (haha)!

Limit your fruit intake depending on the day: high, medium, and low. Factoring in all carbs for the day, ideally one to two servings max could be fruit. Berries are always the best choice because they don't impact your blood sugar as much as many of the other options. If you can, choose raspberries, blackberries, blueberries, and strawberries whenever possible—or always, because I said do damn it! ;P

STARCHES

There is a big difference between regular, leafy green veggies and the starchy kind. Starchy carbs hit the glycemic index much higher than leafy greens and are significantly more calorically dense. They also give off more energy through the digestion process.

There is also a difference between starchy vegetables, like roots and tubers, versus grains. The biggest difference is that grains can cause leaky gut and inflammation. And since inflammation is the number one predecessor to disease, I advise very little to none. I eat zero or very little on extreme occasion. A lot of people can be sensitive to grains without even knowing it, so it is best to stay away from them. If you'd like a good read on grains to understand them better, pick up a book called *Grain Brain: The Surprising Truth about Wheat, Carbs, and Sugar—Your Brain's Silent Killers* by David Perlmutter—very insightful.

Now, on to healthy roots and tubers, which are slow-digesting, not to mention the fiber will help the digestion process remain regular. These keep you fuller longer, and safe starches give you sustained energy throughout the day. Plus, they are packed full of vitamins, minerals, and antioxidants and are very nutrient dense.

Processed Carbohydrates a.k.a. Bad Carbs

Here's a quick and easy way to get on the right track with carb choices. Ask yourself, "Is this carbohydrate processed?" If it's been altered from its natural state in any way, chances are it's a bad carb.

Classic examples of bad carbs include breakfast cereal, sweetened instant oatmeal, tortillas, and white or whole wheat bread and pastas.

Grains are another "no-no," but most people let these slip by. They think as long as it's "whole grain," it's no problem.

Big mistake.

The problem with grains is that the human body doesn't possess the mechanisms to completely break them down.

When you digest gluten or wheat peptides, they force open the tight junctions in the small intestine, which leaves your immune system open to attack. This can lead to inflammation, eventually going on to cause major diseases, including the autoimmune diseases that are becoming so common in today's society.

Stop eating grains and you can avoid many of today's common immune disorders. You'll want to experiment to observe how your body reacts. Remove grains from your diet for a month. My feeling, based on what I have witnessed after working with hundreds of thousands of clients, is that you feel much better, and once (if) you decide to reintroduce them, you will quickly realize why I feel so strongly about eliminating them all together.

What Are Processed Carbs?

Processed carbs are just what they sound like. They are highly processed, manufactured, and/or altered from their natural state. When you think unprocessed, think whole foods from nature, foods you can hunt and gather. Vegetables and fruits you can pick and harvest, animals you can hunt, nuts and seeds you can source in the wild.

In comparison to unprocessed food, processed foods are far less nutritious. In fact, many have zero nutritional value whatsoever.

The closer you eat to nature, the higher the nutrient density, the better you'll feel, the faster you'll lose fat, and the more productive you will become.

In a lot of cases, highly processed diets cause weight gain, diabetes, and heart disease. But the thing most people don't realize, as a result of eating a processed diet for so long, is how it alters the way they feel, as they are just used to feeling "that way," which might not be that good at all. A diet full of processed carbs can have an effect on things like focus, energy, attention, and quality of sleep. Often, people don't realize that this isn't normal because they are so accustomed to the feelings that they are deemed as natural.

Our bodies are amazing at adaptation and after a while, we think it's the norm. I can tell you, based on experience, there is a better life awaiting you the closer you eat to nature and the less refined your diet becomes.

While processed carbs are convenient, they come with some big time tradeoffs. These include chronic inflammation, autoimmune disorders, and metabolic dysfunction, and if you're reading this and you're in your twenties or thirties you likely haven't experienced the effects of this yet. I say yet, because over time and as you get older you will see and feel the ramifications of a poor, highly-processed diet.

Signs That Identify a Highly Processed Diet

There are some pretty easy ways to tell if the food you are eating is processed or not.

For starters, you cannot go and pick or hunt for a donut, a Ho Ho, or a Twinkie. This is one indicator, but there are foods that are much harder to assess. Another good way to begin understanding whether a food is processed is by looking at the nutrition label. What does the ingredient list say? Does it include high fructose corn syrup? How many ingredients are there? These are just a few questions you can ask yourself when considering something that you are unaware of.

A good rule to follow that works most of the time is your foods should have a handful of ingredients or less. Now, there are exceptions to the rule. In this case, Google is your friend. If you cannot pronounce them they are likely not great. Removing processed food from your diet may sound challenging, it's not. Pretend like you are paying detective. (Haha, it works!)

A little tip, start slow by finding substitutes for all of the foods you love. That's what I have done. If you follow me on Snapchat, then you know I eat all of the good stuff made with healthy, whole ingredients. For example, if you love soda, switching to flavored club soda is a good substitute. If you love chocolate like I do, replace the candy bars with some dark chocolate cocoa chips (60% or better). There's a healthy alternative for everything, it took me a while to figure it out, but once you see what's out there you'll feel like I do and will never want to put crappy stuff in your body again.

The biggest benefit comes when you give up processed carbs altogether—the quicker you do, the quicker you will begin to see major differences in your body. You will also notice that you have better, more sustained energy, focus, and drive. Your quality of breath will go up. It's likely you will notice that your mental clarity and cognitive function has improved.

Carbs: Using Them Wisely

CARBOHYDRATE STATUS

PHASE 1: For 7 days—100% of your carbohydrates are going to be sweet potatoes.

PHASE 2: During your Sweet Potato Diet Cycle—100% of your carbohydrates are going to be sweet potatoes in the correct portions for the carb cycle you choose.

AFTER PHASE 1 AND 2: Choose carbohydrates from the approved foods list.

CARBOHYDRATE SOURCES

- Carbohydrates come from four **sources**, such as:
- **Vegetables**, such as spinach, asparagus, and broccoli
- **Fruits**, such as berries, cherries, and kiwi
- Starches & **Tubers**, such as rice, potatoes and turnips
- **Processed sources**, such as flour, HFCS (high fructose corn syrup), table sugar (sucrose), and pasta

Carbs alone will not make you gain weight. The type you eat and the amount you eat are what influences fat mass. That's why the Sweet Potato Diet program focuses on really smart, cutting-edge carb cycling.

Eating the wrong carbs at the wrong time slams the brakes on fat loss.

Eating the right carbs at just the right time will make results soar.

VEGETABLES, FRUITS, AND STARCHES: Eat the right carbs, and you'll be well-fueled for your workouts and energized throughout the day, with a revved-up metabolism that supports fat loss.

Some of the best carbohydrates you can eat include steel cut oats in moderation (a grain), sweet potatoes, quinoa (which is a seed), gluten-free rice cakes, white potatoes (if you aren't a fan of sweet potatoes), and white rice. Many people will question eating white rice, but trust me, I have done plenty of research and the germ found in brown rice is extremely susceptible to rancidity, which is bad because of the very high content of polyunsaturated fat it contains; this is easily oxidized and leads to all sorts of problematic reactions in the body.

If you absolutely can't live without bread, a great substitute is Ezekiel bread, a sprouted grain. Of course, the Sweet Potato Diet is designed to help you simplify all of this by replacing all of the right carbs with the best carb, sweet potatoes. And, even if you don't know how to enjoy sweet potatoes right now, there are a ton of recipes in this book to help you find a dish for your taste.

CARBOHYDRATES (SIMPLE VS. COMPLEX)

All carbohydrates fall into two different categories: simple and complex. Simple carbohydrates are made of short molecular chains containing oxygen, carbon, and hydrogen. Simple carbs are easily digested and very quickly increase blood sugar levels. Examples are foods like bananas, dried fruit, 100% fruit juice, and honey. The World Health Organization lists sugar (glucose and fructose) and other simple carbohydrates as leading factors of obesity. They are also associated with tooth decay, type 2 diabetes, cardiovascular disease, and breast cancer. However, not all simple carbohydrates are bad for you all the time.

Complex carbohydrates, such as leafy green vegetables and potatoes, are healthier than simple carbs because they contain vitamins, minerals, and antioxidants. Examples of some complex carbohydrates that are good include sweet potatoes (of course!), white rice, quinoa, white potatoes, and then for fruit, apples, grapes, berries, and grapefruit are among the best.

UNDERSTANDING SIMPLE SUGARS

GLUCOSE: the most basic and most easily used sugar. It's broken down from starches, such as potatoes, rice, and quinoa.

FRUCTOSE: found in fruit and is preferential to the liver, not skeletal muscle.

LACTOSE: the sugar found in dairy, which is broken down into glucose and galactose. It can be a problem for some people.

HIGH FRUCTOSE CORN SYRUP (HFCS): an unhealthy, synthetic, processed sweetener that can lead to weight gain and should be avoided.

OTHER SIMPLE SUGARS: maltose, dextrose, maltodextrin.

You don't need to overthink simple sugars. This is just to give you a basic understanding.

Proteins: The Most Essential Nutrient

Proteins are one of the most important elements of any diet.

They are the "building blocks" for your organs, muscles, bones, blood, skin, enzymes, hormones, and more. Even your hair and nails are made with protein. Proteins (just like fats and carbohydrates) also provide energy (calories) for your body to burn. However, we want you to think of protein as the calories that are the building blocks (the frame of the car) and fats and carbohydrates as the fuel which you use to go (power the car). The better the protein, the stronger and more durable the frame. The better the fat and carbohydrates, the more efficiently you travel and the longer the car will run without major tune-ups (in our case hospital visits).

Essential for Everyone, Including Women

Protein is essential for *everyone*. Man, woman, young, old, training or not, you *need* protein.

Women often don't get enough protein because they think it will make them big and bulky. I want to reassure you that's not the case.

Women simply don't possess the hormones necessary to pack on lots of muscle mass. It would take years and years of hard work to gain appreciable muscle, and often a number of other "supplements," which I'll never recommend. In fact, protein intake helps women to achieve a slender, more lean body.

BENEFITS OF PROTEIN

Everyone needs protein. It's not just for athletes.

- Protein increases the metabolism for faster fat loss
- It helps repair and grow muscle
- It promotes satiety, helping you feel fuller from meals
- Protein helps with fat storage and release
- It helps with necessary displacement of carb ratio

METABOLISM AND THE THERMIC EFFECT OF FOOD (TEF)

Protein is a very costly macronutrient for the body to metabolize. This means your body actually burns calories in order to digest protein. From a fat-loss perspective, it makes sense to include protein with every meal.

Without sufficient protein in your diet, you begin losing muscle mass as you age, which results in a slower metabolic rate, making fat loss an even greater challenge.

REPAIRING SKELETAL MUSCLE AND TISSUE

Training and day-to-day physical activity create consistent micro-damage to the body's muscles and tendons. Protein plays a major role in repairing the damage, providing the building blocks for the repair of tissue.

SATIETY

Satiety is essentially how full you feel after eating. Fat, carbs, and protein all affect hormonal secretion (and satiety) differently. But protein is king.

Protein's molecular structure means it takes longer for the body to break down than carbohydrates. Furthermore, it's very hard to overeat protein because it's so filling.

FAT STORAGE AND FAT RELEASE

Without getting too complicated, it's important for you to understand a couple of hormones: insulin and glucagon. Together, these hormones regulate blood sugar. Animal-based sources of protein are very dense with amino acids, and create a greater secretion of glucagon, the "fat release" hormone. Insulin is the master "fat storage" hormone. When it comes to losing fat, it is "fat release" you're after. While beans, nuts, and dairy contain protein, the quantity and quality of protein is substandard at best. That's why it's best to eat animal-based complete proteins.

DISPLACING THE CARBOHYDRATE RATIO

Typically, if your protein intake is high, your carb intake will be lower. And when this ratio is dominated by animal-based protein, fats naturally fall into place and carbs can be easily portioned and adjusted based on your additional needs.

DAILY PROTEIN RECOMMENDATION

- Consume protein with every meal.
- If you are eating the recommended palm-sized amount of quality protein at each meal, you will be getting enough for your body mass. Your palm is proportionate to your body, and those with larger builds and larger hands will naturally eat more protein than those with smaller builds and smaller hands.

PROTEIN SOURCES

There are many possible sources of protein for your diet, including legumes (beans), dairy, nuts, and seeds.

However, you should focus on animal-based protein such as:

- Beef
- Fish
- Chicken
- Pork
- Eggs

PROTEIN TIPS FOR FAT LOSS

Preparation

Prepare more protein when you cook and use leftovers as snacks. Simply toss half of a chicken breast into a ziploc bag so you can quickly grab it out of the fridge for breakfast or as a snack later in the day.

Cottage Cheese and Plain Non-fat Greek Yogurt

Cottage cheese and plain non-fat Greek yogurt are very high in protein (Greek yogurt contains nearly twice the amount of protein as "regular" yogurt, with roughly half the calories). Their thick, filling consistency helps you feel full, helping you to avoid hunger pangs and food cravings. These are to be eaten in moderation.

Fish

Besides being an excellent source of dietary protein, oily fish (trout, salmon, mackeral) is beneficial because of its omega-3 fatty acid content. Omega-3 fatty acids support good heart health and are essential for your brain and nervous system.

The American Heart Association says that omega-3 fatty acids decrease your risk of abnormal heartbeats, lower your blood pressure, and decrease plaque buildup (which can lead to strokes). The recommendation is to eat at least two servings of fish each week.

Pea and Rice Protein

Pea and rice proteins are good sources of protein for vegetarians and vegans only.

Beef Jerky

The quality of beef jerky can vary a great deal. Look for jerky that does not contain high fructose corn syrup (HFCS). Despite media attention about sodium nitrate, it's not a concern.

Protein Powder

Until your whole foods have been dialed in, I suggest avoiding protein powder altogether, and that's coming from someone who sells it. It's unnecessary and I'd rather you focus your time, energy, and money on real, natural foods. I use grass-fed protein "Morellifit Nutrition," of course, to supplement protein between meals, but never in place of my protein in my meals. However, it will be discussed later in the section on supplements.

Protein Bars

As far as nutrient quality is concerned, protein bars are NOT the best choice. The few bars on the market that are actually okay are usually much more expensive, portion for portion, than real-food sources of protein. That said, a protein bar in some instances is better than nothing. All processed bars still have some drawbacks and become a concern when eaten on a regular basis.

If you must eat a protein bar, be sure to check that all the ingredients are natural, and there are no harmful chemical sweeteners or fillers. Bars like this are out there; they are just harder to find and require you to closely read the labels. The best choice is making your own. There's lots of good recipes out there.

Breakfast MUST Contain Protein

The typical North American breakfast of milk, cereal, and juice is loaded with sugar and carbs and has very little protein and no good fats. Eggs are KING for breakfast because of their huge biological protein value (BPV). Protein first thing in the morning stimulates your body's use of fat for fuel and stops muscle loss.

Fats: More Essential Than You Think

Despite all of the mixed messages you may have picked up from the mass market diet industry over the years, fat doesn't make you fat. While fat is calorically dense at 9 calories per gram, it doesn't spike inulin. This is important because insulin spikes can tell the body to store fat, and you don't want that.

KNOW YOUR FATS

The human body needs dietary fats. That's why you'll hear me referring to fats as "essential."

Our bodies and central nervous systems require fats for recovery. Fats are an integral part of hormonal balance, hormonal regulation, and repair at the cellular level.

Fats are composed of fatty acids and glycerol and help generate hormones in the body as well as prostaglandins (hormone-like substances). This all means fats are key to a number of incredible processes in our bodies, such as:

- Constriction and dilation of vascular smooth muscle cells
- Regulation of inflammation
- Control of calcium movement in and out of bone cells
- Control of cell growth
- Transmission of signals to the kidney to increase filtration rates
- Regulation of hormones

If your diet is too low in healthy essential fats (from the proper sources—I'll get to that in a bit), your body runs the risk of being low in prostaglandins, and your hormones don't function as they should. This will actually work against you, slowing down your fat loss (if not stopping it entirely). Fats are a major key to fat loss.

Testosterone is another really important hormone for fat loss—and not just for men. Healthy testosterone levels are critical for women choosing to live a lean lifestyle, too. Dietary fat maintains higher testosterone levels, which help both men and women to:

- Stay lean (because testosterone supports lean muscle mass)
- Build muscle and burn fat
- Gain strength from workouts
- Maintain a healthy libido

Dietary fats from natural healthy sources provide fat soluble vitamins (vitamins A, D, E, and K), which help to:

- Regulate processes such as blood clotting
- Provide antioxidant support
- Improve skin, hair, and nail health

And we love dietary fats because they're tasty, satisfying, and filling. Just adding 5–10 grams of healthy fat to your meals (not snacks) will help you stay satisfied for hours.

But before we get too carried away with just how awesome healthy fats are, a word of caution. At 9 calories per gram, fats are the most energy-dense macronutrient and can be quite easy to overeat. You need to eat fat—just be cautious and practice good portion control.

THE 4 TYPES OF FAT

1. **POLYUNSATURATED FATTY ACIDS (PUFA)** found in fish, flax, canola, and other industrialized seed oils. Polyunsaturated fatty acids (PUFAs) oxidize (become rancid) easily. This means they can either be inflammatory (omega-6), or anti-inflammatory (omega-3). You can consume PUFAs, but be aware that they become unstable when exposed to heat and/or oxygen.

2. **MONOUNSATURATED FATTY ACIDS (MUFA)** found in olive oil, some nuts (macadamias), and avocados. The fatty acid profile in red meat is 50% monounsaturated fats (MUFAs).

3. **SATURATED FATTY ACIDS (SFA)** found in coconut and animals. These are essential for testosterone production and have wrongly been accused of being unhealthy. A higher intake of saturated fatty acids is great for optimal hormonal secretion.

4. **TRANS FATTY ACIDS (TFA)**, despite being demonized by the media, are not all bad. Naturally occurring trans fatty acids, such as conjugated linoleic acid (CLA) and vaccenic acid, have huge benefits for fat loss and maintaining muscle.

INFLAMMATION, YOUR FAT LOSS ENEMY

Inflammation happens to even the healthiest people. In fact, it's the body's natural response to stress, including the stress of intense exercise.

But it can be your worst enemy when it comes to fat loss. The Sweet Potato Diet is going to teach you how to control inflammation to ensure it doesn't get in the way of your fat loss goals.

Inflammation can be a result of:

- Excessive training
- Chronic stress
- Lack of sleep
- Poor dietary choices

One of the biggest dietary offenders is linoleic acid (LA), an omega-6 fatty acid found in foods such as:

- Grains
- Pastas
- Breads
- Seed oils (safflower, corn, soy, and nuts)

Studies have shown that excessive consumption of omega-6 fats can increase your risk for heart disease, depression, arthritis, diabetes, cancer, and many other health issues.

I suggest eating nuts (see grocery list), but be aware that regular store-bought nuts are usually roasted in oil, which damages the fats in the nuts. Macadamias are the best choice: they have monounsaturated fats (MUFAs) and saturated fatty acids (SFAs). Always look for "dry roasted" or raw nuts.

COCONUT OIL AND REAL BUTTER'S SURPRISING BENEFITS

If you are already cooking with coconut oil, you're one step ahead of most people.

This fat's medium-chain triglycerides (MCT) are preferential for energy production versus energy storage, thus making it useful in longer training sessions, especially when glycogen capacity is an issue.

Another amazing source of dietary fat is real butter, preferably grass-fed. It's great for gastrointestinal (GI) health and digestion, among other things.

WHAT ABOUT ANIMAL FATS?

Fats from animals are commonly thought of as all saturated fat.

And with all the bad publicity, most people stay away from them.

I like to look at animal fats a little differently, taking into account how today's meat is raised. Red meat is generally 50% monounsaturated fats (MUFAs) and 50% saturated fat (SFA), with the saturated fat containing very high amounts of extremely healthy, naturally occurring conjugated linoleic acid (CLA) and vaccenic acid (VA).

As a result of what most of today's chickens are fed (grains), the birds store fat as omega-6 polyunsaturated fatty acids (PUFAs). Yes, the ones we try to avoid in large doses. This is why I often choose red meat (grass-fed whenever possible) over chicken (vegetable fed). I am not suggesting that you shouldn't eat chicken (I eat a lot); just make sure it's not your only source of animal protein.

In fact, it's critical that you vary your protein sources.

Pork is another great choice, as long as it's from a quality source. Bacon fat is 50% saturated fat (SFA); it's healthy and won't oxidize. Use it as you would butter. Often I cook my eggs in it. Throw in some sweet potatoes for a little starch and now we are talking. Delicious.

ARGUABLY THE TWO BEST FATS

Two of my go-to sources of healthy fats are avocados and extra virgin olive oil, which are great for supporting hormones and fueling beyond your glycogen stores. And these whole foods are chock full of micronutrients and fat-soluble vitamins. Not to mention avocados are one of nature's top superfoods with a laundry list of health benefits. They are a staple in our home, our kids at two and four absolutely love them. They make it to almost every plate.

FATTY ACIDS IN FISH

Fish is important, but you need to eat the right kind of fish. In most cases, store-bought fish is crap due to the diet of grains farmed fish are fed. Choose to get "wild" caught fish whenever possible, as it holds far more nutritional value and a much better fatty acid profile.

I'll discuss supplementing with fish oil (which I recommend, by the way) in the Supplement section of *The Sweet Potato Diet*. Flaxseed, linseed, flax oil, and chia seeds are other sources of omega-6 polyunsaturated fatty acids. However, the conversion from alpha linolenic acid (ALA) to eicosapentaenoic acid (EPA) and docosahexaenoic acid (DHA) is poor, so I don't recommend them over fish oil as a primary source of EPA and DHA.

The Problem of Food Intolerances and Sensitivities

We probably all eat something once in a while that doesn't agree with us. For some people this is an occasional thing, resulting in a little indigestion. For others, food allergies and intolerances can pose very real threats to health and fat loss.

It's important that you become aware of how food affects your body and makes you feel.

Here's a simple tracking system for you to use during your transition into the Sweet Potato Diet's healthy eating plan:

1. As you eat a particular food or meal, think about how it makes you feel.

2. If you feel good after the meal or food, place a smiley face next to it.

3. If you feel bad or sluggish after the meal or food, place a frowning face next to it.

4. This system sounds super simple.

But what you're doing is beginning to investigate possible food sensitivities and intolerances. You'll soon become very aware of your body's relationship with individual foods.

You may wonder why you should bother with food intolerances and sensitivities if you're only dieting for aesthetics or to lose fat. There are actually two very good reasons for anyone to root out food intolerances.

REASON 1: CHRONIC INFLAMMATION

Certain foods might cause you to experience low-grade, chronic inflammation that is not only harmful to your health, but also robs your body of important nutritional resources.

If your body is using precious macronutrients, micronutrients, and minerals to repair damaged tissue from a food intolerance or sensitivity, then it's not recovering from any training or exercise as well as it could be, and it's possibly even not building lean body mass or burning fat.

REASON 2: CORTISOL AND STRESS

Some foods can contribute to cortisol release and secondary stress.

Think of an extremely sensitive celiac (gluten intolerant) person. Even a small amount of gluten can result in major sickness for that individual due to the release of hormones such as epinephrine and cortisol. It's important for all of us to control these inflammatory stress hormones, even if you think you're not actually intolerant to the food.

Be mindful of the following common inflammatory foods:

- Peppers, white potatoes, oats, eggplant, and tomatoes. The glycoalkaloids found in these foods can lead to inflammation.
- Beans and other legumes. If you consume these foods at all, always make sure they are thoroughly cooked and pre-soaked when necessary.
- Dairy in all forms (cheese, milk, whey, casein, and yogurt). Try to keep dairy consumption to a very minimum.

While I realize this may be difficult if any of these foods are favorites or staples in your diet, I've provided solid substitutes for you in the accompanying Sweet Potato Diet Approved Food List & Grocery Guide.

PART 2

THE CARB CYCLING PHASE

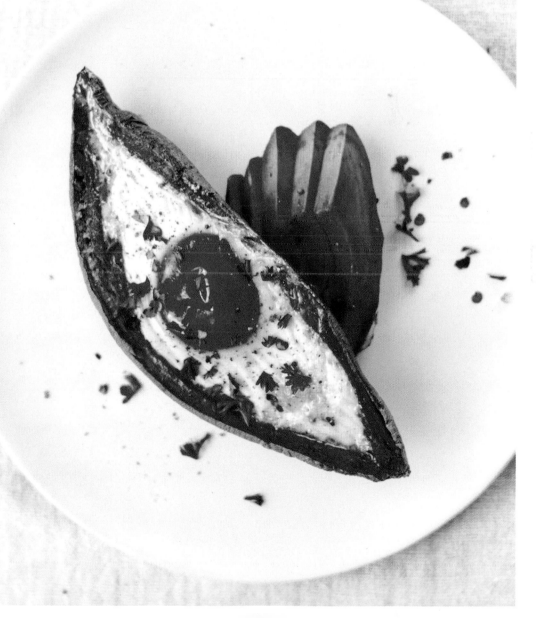

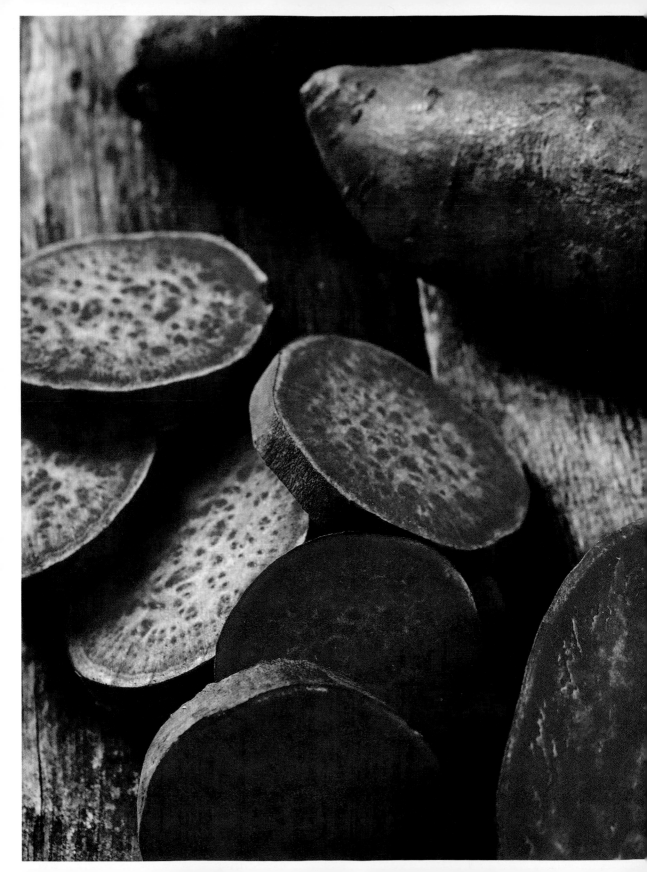

CHAPTER 4:

The Science of Super Carb Cycling

t's crazy to look back after all of the diets I have tried in the past, I would have never thought as I tried and failed, tried and failed, diet after diet that I would go on to write the diet book that trumps them all. The science of carb cycling combined with the nutritional power of the sweet potato has allowed me to change more lives than I could even imagine.

You see, if you're like me, then you've tried plenty of diets and have been left disappointed on many occasions. All of the false promises create a new sense of hope, and then it all comes crashing down pound after pound, more often than not ending up in a place worse than when you started.

I can assure you that when you follow the blueprint I have laid out for you in the upcoming chapters, you will drop body fat and carve out a body you never even knew you had. You don't have to hope or wish anymore, you need to simply follow the plan because it has worked tens of thousands of times. The proof is in the pudding—and I have a whole lot of pudding.

Before I put all of your carb-cycling concerns to rest, let me first tell you what carb cycling is, why it works so effectively, and how we are going to use it to manipulate your macros just enough to shock your body into serious fat loss.

Go grab your sweet potatoes because here's where it gets fun!

What Exactly Is Carb Cycling?

Carb cycling is a way of eating that rotates between low-carbohydrate days and high-carbohydrate days. During each week, we manipulate carbs from high to low so your body never knows what to expect. This ensures that your metabolism never has an opportunity to adapt, which means results for you. When carbs are high, fats (the other energy source) are low, and when carbs are low, fats are higher with protein staying consistent for the most part.

You see, it's all about the cycle you choose (I give you three), and the beauty is that you can continue to get results by changing the cycle. Think of it like this, low-carb days are deficit days or fat-burning days. This is where you eat below your energy expenditure. The opposite is true for your high-carb days, these are the days where you're in a surplus or in an anabolic state.

The more anabolic days, the more weight (usually muscle) you gain, and the more fat-burning days in the cycle, the more body fat you drop. Now, it's deeper than that because these days work in conjunction to give you the best of both worlds, but for the sake of simplicity it's two days doing two different things. I explain in more detail in the next section.

The secret though is you need both, you cannot have just a bunch of low-carb days because, as you know if you've been paying attention, your body always adapts to the conditions you impose and so it will flatline on low carbs across the board.

Carb cycling rides on the success of low-carb days but combines them with metabolism-boosting, higher-carb days, so your body keeps burning fat. The high-carb days fuel the furnace, get it nice and hot, then you drop it like it's hot (haha I always wanted to say that). No really, you drop your carbs and because your furnace is scorching hot you burn fat. That's the power of carb cycling! Burn baby burn. Can you tell I am excited?!

I am excited because I have seen this power in full effect, in my own transformation and countless others. And let's face it, how long can you eat little to no carbs? That's exactly why most people struggle with low-carbohydrate diets, finding them restrictive and hard to follow. Carb cycling solves this problem with its inferno-driving high-carb days and reward meals.

Carb cycling is a proven strategy for fat loss and is the best way to reach your goal. Once you've reached your first goal, you can choose a different cycle to continue winning at weight loss (which I'll reveal to you later in the book).

Why Cycle Carbs?

Your metabolism is an amazing system of biochemical processes that work around the clock to keep you alive and well. Whether you are awake or asleep, active or resting, your metabolism is always working.

When your body is working off a high level of carbohydrates, it is in an "anabolic state." This means it is growing new cells and building tissues, growing muscle, and strengthening bones. All of these are anabolic activities.

When your body is not in an anabolic state, it is in a "fat-burning state," breaking down complex molecules into simpler ones to release energy. When we eat, our body breaks down nutrients so they can be used as energy.

At any given time, our bodies fluctuate between these two states in a delicate balance that allows us to produce the energy our bodies need to live and grow.

Carb cycling is really smart, purposefully driving your body into alternating states of anabolic and fat-burning activity. Carbohydrates fuel anabolic activity, so on your high-carb days you'll be building muscle and increasing your metabolism. On lower-carb days, your body will be catapulted into a fat-burning state, and the energy your body needs will come primarily from stored fat.

Smart, huh? This is how carb cycling melts away stored fat and helps get you leaner all while preserving lean muscle tissue. You'll turn your body into a fat-burning machine, and the result is continual fat loss, with absolutely no diet plateaus. And just in case one does show (because everyone is different), we've got something for that, too. Stay tuned!

Fuel for Your Furnace

First things first. Your body is like a furnace, which needs to burn fuel in order to function. Your body's fuel is the calories in your food.

Through the process of digestion, your body transforms the food (calories) into usable energy. Then, it expends that energy in various activities, including cellular activity, recovery, and actual workouts. This is a process that is ongoing all day, every day.

And here's where the formula comes in…

If you take in more calories than you burn, your body will turn the excess energy into stores of fat, so it can survive when food is scarce. You will gain weight.

If you take in the same number of calories your body burns, your weight will remain consistent.

Lastly, if you take in fewer calories than you burn, your body will use stored fat to burn as energy, and you will lose weight.

Simple, right?

Not quite.

So, now let's talk about metabolism and its role in weight loss.

The Metabolic Effect

Some people have difficulty losing weight because they don't understand how their body's metabolism works. Let's make sure you're never one of them.

Your metabolism is designed to protect you against starvation. So, as long as your body is receiving fuel (food) in sufficient quantity and at regular intervals, it will instinctively know that calories are plentiful. No need to panic and store fat. Your body will "rev up" its metabolic furnace and burn fuel efficiently.

But if your body is not receiving adequate fuel to function properly, it will "cool down," and the rate of your metabolism will slow. This is a great way to conserve energy, allowing your body to save fuel. Can you imagine what this means for weight loss?

People who want to lose weight often make the mistake of eating less food, less often. But what they just don't realize is that they are actually working against their bodies. When you take away the fuel your body needs, your body goes into "starvation mode" and begins to slow down. It doesn't think there is any more fuel coming...at least not for a while. And if this happens while you are attempting to lose weight, your progress stalls or comes to a complete stop altogether.

I want you to avoid fat-loss frustration and plateaus. That's why I designed the Sweet Potato Diet. It always works with your metabolism, never against it. Here's how we are going to speed up your metabolism.

- Eat frequently
- Eat carbohydrates
- Build muscle
- Exercise consistently

EAT FREQUENTLY

Most people are used to eating three meals a day, anything from four to six hours apart. Eating regularly and frequently (every three hours) stimulates your metabolism, helps reduce cravings and hunger pangs, and keeps your digestive system stimulated and active, all of which burn more energy.

EAT CARBOHYDRATES

Eating complex carbohydrates helps you lose weight in a few ways. First, they keep your metabolism burning calories. If you deplete your body of the fuel it wants and needs, it will naturally slow your metabolism down to meet the new standards you are setting. And that is the opposite of what we want. Second, complex carbs fill you up and burn slowly, which keeps you feeling fuller, longer. These complex carbs help you feel less hungry and help you avoid cravings. Finally, they also help regulate your blood sugar and insulin levels. (Remember how important the master hormone is to your fat loss?)

BUILD MUSCLE

Building more muscle will definitely help you lose body fat. Gaining muscle boosts your resting metabolic rate because your body demands more calories to maintain muscle than fat, which means you'll be able to eat more and more, not less and less like most starvation diets.

Not to mention, building muscle has several other advantages. It encourages your body to burn fat stores rather than muscle tissue when you are losing weight and helps to slow the muscle loss that comes naturally with the aging process. Muscle also helps protect your bones, regulates blood sugar levels, and helps you to rest. Do you notice how I say "lose fat" instead of lose weight? That's because we don't ever want to sacrifice muscle for the sake of fat, we want to drop body fat alone and keep our muscle. Let's be specific, it's the fat we don't want, and muscle eats fat, so let's not lose any of that.

EXERCISE

Exercise is essential to maintaining a healthy body, whether you are choosing to lose fat or not. Our bodies were designed to move. Make regular exercise an important part of your Sweet Potato

Diet plan. It will stimulate your body to burn additional calories, help you to build some lean muscle tissue, reduce stress, elevate your mood, and even help you to sleep better.

There is a section on exercise, providing you with easy, at-home exercises designed to help get you moving. With our simple-to-follow guide, you will be burning calories right in your home in just a few minutes a day.

OK, so now that you have some context around carb cycling and an understanding as to how your metabolic furnace works, let's get into some of the specifics.

HOW DO I CHOOSE FROM THE DIFFERENT CARB CYCLES?

Excellent question: I devoted an entire chapter to it. Take a look at the upcoming chapter "Three Cycles." It will give you everything you need to select the right carb cycle for you. If you've never carb cycled before, I suggest starting with the first cycle (simple).

HOW SHOULD I STRUCTURE MY TRAINING AROUND THE CYCLE?

Knowing how to combine workouts and nutrition is what will bring you mind-blowing results from the Sweet Potato Diet. Read the chapter "Structuring Your Workouts Around the Cycle," which tells you exactly how to make your carb cycle and training work together for even more effective results.

HOW DO I CALCULATE MY DAILY CARB INTAKE?

It's critical that you properly portion your carb intake for each of the four types of carb days. Fail to pay attention to these quick and easy portioning methods and you won't be carb cycling the Sweet Potato Diet way. Use the chapter "Four Types of Carb Days" and stick to your portion sizes. You'll learn how to understand the difference between each type of day and how to measure carb intake in a matter of minutes.

WHAT EXACTLY DO I EAT ON THE SWEET POTATO DIET?

Nutrition is the foundation upon which the Sweet Potato Diet is built. You're going to find at least a few chapters that discuss approved foods, nutrition timing, grocery lists, and meal choices in this book.

Remember to use your approved foods list, grocery guide, and recipe guide. They are amazing resources which make it super easy for you to shop for, plan, and prepare your meals. It's all done for you.

HOW MANY MEALS DO I EAT ON THE SWEET POTATO DIET?

The answer is five, and while I know for some of you that may seem like a lot, you just have to trust me. All you can do is your best, if you continue to do just that, nothing more, I can assure you will be eating five meals spaced out every few hours in no time. Remember that furnace is going to be burning fat again in no time.

Your goal is to eat meals spaced every three hours from within one hour of waking up. This helps regulate insulin levels, keeps you from getting hungry, and helps to balance the hormone cortisol (remember, high cortisol levels can lead to weight gain.) Follow the portions in your carb cycle, drink plenty of water, and very quickly you'll realize this is the way it should have been a long time ago. Make sure you drink your water (reference back to the beginning if you don't remember). This will help digestion and make your new eating habits easier.

WHEN DO I GET TO CHEAT?

Ok, let's not call it "cheat"—rather "reward." I mean isn't that what you're doing? You're rewarding yourself for sticking to the diet. But, you only get to do so one out of every ten meals and it must replace one of your meals on your high-carb day. Let me explain. You have to eat according to the plan (not even 1% variance) for nine total meals, then on the tenth you get to reward yourself with a meal of your choice. If the tenth meal falls on a low carb day, wait until the next high-carb day to enjoy your meal. I also suggest planning your reward meals on days where you are post-active, the more active you are, the less likely you are to gain body fat during this surplus.

I believe whole heartedly in reward meals. Most people need the freedom and flexibility of knowing they can deviate from a clean diet once in a while, and what better way to use it than a reward for consistency and progress.

You don't have to reward yourself on this diet, it's entirely up to you. For those of you who decide to be a bit flexible, use the 90/10 rule. Remember, consistency is key to success with the Sweet Potato Diet. Minor deviations won't cause everything to come crashing down, as long as you stay consistent 90% of the time or better.

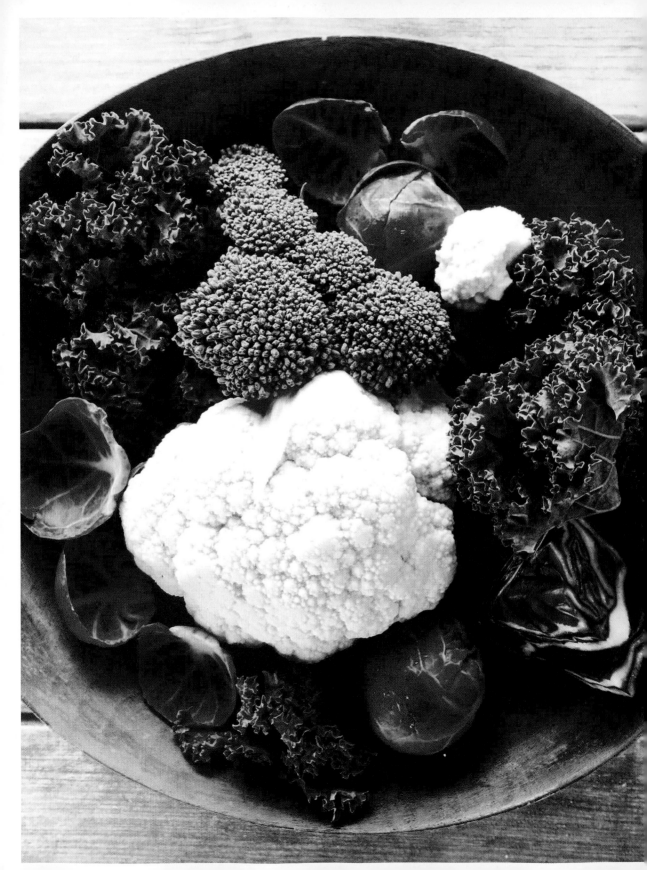

CHAPTER 5:

Four Super Carb Days

Four Types of "Carb Days"

There are four different types of carb days when breaking down how to work each of the carb cycles. Each type of day differs not only in the amount of carbs, but in the amount of protein and fats as well to keep things balanced.

You'll need to understand the four different types of carb days, how to calculate your carb intake for each day, and what to eat. Then, you apply this knowledge to the carb cycle you choose in the next chapter. Don't worry, it's super easy and I will walk you through it.

If you need additional support, you can visit SweetPotatoDiet.com or catch me on Twitter @morellifit.

HIGH-CARB DAYS

Your high-carb days are loaded with healthy, carbohydrate-rich sweet potatoes.

In fact, you may find that you are eating more carbohydrates on these days than you typically ate on your regular diet. Trust me on this. If you want to see success, these scheduled high-carb days are vital. Don't make the mistake of lowering your carbs on high-carb days because it will be counterproductive and slow your progress.

By boosting your consumption of carbs on these days, you'll get a metabolic and leptin spike that will help you feel your best throughout the entire cycle and lose fat at a faster rate.

What to Eat

Your high-carb days should focus on including a protein and a carbohydrate at every meal. The combination of these two ingredients will stimulate your body to build muscle and burn energy. Over time, the result will be a leaner body and high metabolism.

Vegetables are always a great part of a balanced and nutrient-rich meal, but on high-carb days it's okay to go lighter on them. The emphasis on these days is to feed your body high concentrations of muscle-building, energy-burning fuel.

Focus your carbohydrate intake on these days around the sweet potato. Fruit can be added, if you must, but keep it to just 1 serving.

Less Fat

Your fat intake on high-carb days will be lowest. This is because you will be getting most of your calories from carbohydrates and protein. As carbs go down for each type of day, the fats rise in proportion.

Avoid the Binge

Eating a lot of carbs can make you want to eat even more carbs, and it can be hard to stop yourself. Stick to the protocol. The longer you are on the Sweet Potato Diet, the less this will happen. Remember, you can always eat more veggies if you get hungry.

MEDIUM-CARB DAYS

Your medium-carb days will be more similar to traditional diets where your carbohydrate intake is set at a normal level.

What to Eat

Since you aren't eating as many carbohydrates on these days, you'll want to eat a mixture of starchy sweet potatoes and non-starchy carbohydrates, leafy greens, and a serving of approved fruit if you'd like. Leafy greens don't count against your daily carb consumption. And fruit can help to keep hunger levels lower on your medium-carb days, as liver glycogen (replenished by the fructose in fruit) can help contribute to how hungry you feel. Berries are lower in carbs and sugar, a perfect choice on these days.

Little More *Fat*

Your fat goes up slightly on the medium-carb days. Make sure to increase your fat intake slightly. As carbs go down for each type of day, the fats rise in proportion.

LOW-CARB DAYS

Your low-carb days will be about half the amount of carbs as your high carb days. This is likely much lower than what you are normally eating for carbohydrates on a regular basis. One way to stay successful is that if you find yourself feeling hungry on a low-carb day, you can increase your protein and veggies for the day. Do not eat any fruit whatsoever on your low-carb days.

What to Eat

The carbs on these days should be sweet potatoes, vegetables, and no fruit. Your meals should include a protein, vegetables, and fats. (This is where you make up for not having as many vegetables on high-carb days.) Meals still include protein, so your body continues to build muscle and won't use muscle for fuel. The vegetables provide much-needed vitamins, minerals, and nutrients, and a larger portion of healthy fat alleviates cravings. On low-carb days, the main goal is to get your body to use stored fat to fuel itself.

More *Fat*

Your fat goes up again this time a bit more sharply to make up for only some of the energy you'd get from the carbs on your high-and medium-carb days.

NO-CARB DAYS

As the name implies, your no-carb days consist of **zero carbs**. However, you can and should still enjoy your non-starchy vegetable carbohydrates. In fact, on this day you should turn into a rabbit (haha)! I am not gonna lie, these are the tough days reserved for only the accelerated cycle. I don't recommend choosing the accelerated cycle if you've never carb cycled before. PS: I usually do nothing on these days.

What to Eat

Do not skip your veggies, aka "free carbs," on the no-carb days. You will feel a lot better eating fibrous vegetables on no-carb days because they supply important nutrients and minerals necessary for feeling your best. Increase your protein a bit if you need to, too.

Drinking

Be sure to drink even more water on the no-carb days. And don't worry about needing to urinate more frequently on no- and low-carb days. It's normal, as your body starts to shed excess water weight that it has been hanging on to because you have become more regular.

Most Fat

Boost your dietary fat intake even more. This day should be the day where you consume the highest amount of healthy fats, however, don't go overboard either—otherwise, you'll just defeat the purpose (and results) of the carb cycling approach. We will go over the correct portions for proteins, fats, and carbs in the next section.

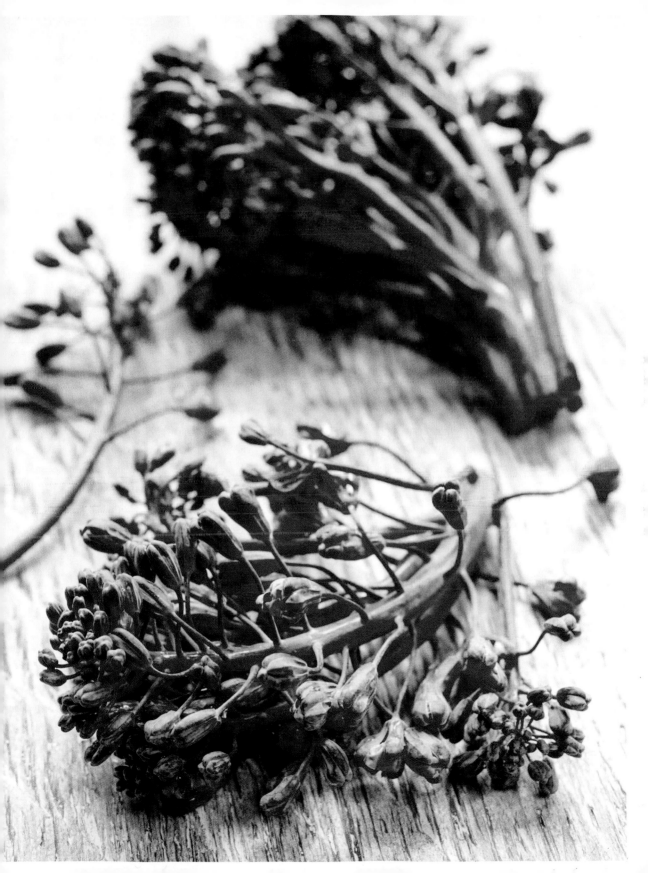

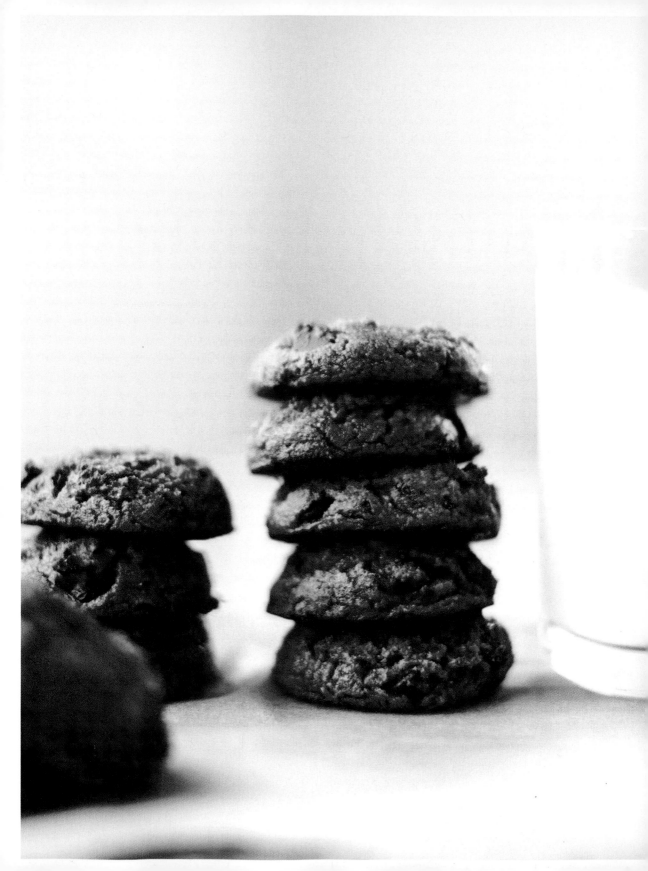

CHAPTER 6:

Three Fat-Burning Cycles and Portioning Your Super Carb Cycle Meals

Three Fat-Burning Cycles

Once you're ready to begin carb cycling, you'll choose from three different carb cycle options:

- **CYCLE OPTION #1—QUICK FIRE CYCLE**—It's highly recommended if you've never carb cycled before that you start here.

- **CYCLE OPTION #2—ACTIVATE HOT CYCLE**—Once you've done the "Quick Fire Cycle" for at least thirty days you are free to move to this cycle. My advice is to stick with the Quick Fire Cycle until your results start to slow down. For some, this could be 6 months or more.

- **CYCLE OPTION #3—ACCELERATED INFERNO CYCLE**—Once you've completed both the Quick Fire and Activate Hot Cycles for at least thirty days each, you are free to move onto this cycle. My advice is to stay in the Activate Hot Cycle for as long as you can, only making the switch once your results have really begun to slow down.

Each cycle is slightly more advanced than the one before, so keep this in mind when choosing the cycle that's right for you. They get harder and harder with the addition of more low- and no-carb days. It's much easier to fall off during these cycles if you haven't experienced carb cycling before. Remember, we are after sustained results. You will drop body fat very quickly no matter which cycle you choose, the idea is to stay the course. Please follow my advice here. I have set this diet to work for you forever. The beauty of this is after you've finished each of these cycles, you can start over shocking your metabolism yet again. It's important that when you're in a cycle you complete at least thirty days. Remember, I told you this was the very last diet book you'll ever have to buy. Crap! That means I can't write another diet book—haha!

Reward Meal

One of the most dangerous pitfalls in your weight-loss and body-transformation journey is likely food cravings and your emotional attachment to food. If you deprive yourself for too long, cravings can swoop in and derail you. I already knew this, so guess what? I have built in reward meals for those of you who need them.

The Sweet Potato Diet has a "reward meal" built into every cycle.

Each of the three carb cycles is designed to offset food cravings with a weekly reward meal.

For reward meals, eat whatever you wish. In fact, I encourage you to eat foods you've been craving so you get the psychological benefits of being able to really enjoy "your favorite" meal every week throughout the entire program.

Just make sure you don't turn your "reward meal" into a binge meal. The only way this meal will slow progress is if you go overboard or haven't followed your carb cycle to the T. And then remember what I said, if that's the case, then no soup for you! LOL. You get no reward meal if you veer off the carb cycle even 1%, that's the deal!

THE REWARD MEAL RULE

You MUST have your reward meal outside of your home. Don't bring these foods into your house. This helps you to stay on track without being unnecessarily tempted, and no left overs whatsoever! Got it? Good.

Here's a neat thing about reward meals. As you progress in your weight loss program, you will likely find your food cravings shift to healthier options or eventually disappear altogether. As your body becomes accustomed to eating healthier foods and less sugar, you will find that your old cravings haunt you less and less.

Cycle Option #1 – Quick Fire Cycle

The Sweet Potato Diet's Quick Fire Cycle is ideal for diet beginners or for those who have never experienced carb cycling before. The Quick Fire Cycle has three low-carb days. For that reason, it's not as challenging. But don't worry, challenging and fat loss aren't positively correlated here, trust me. The three low-carb days have at least one medium- or high-carb day between them. This allows you to enjoy eating more carbs the next day. Keep something in mind, adjust the cycle days to the days of the week where you will thrive best. For example, it might be wise to have your high-carb (reward meal) day on a weekend.

CYCLE PROTOCOL:

DAY 1: High-Carb Day

DAY 2: Medium-Carb Day

DAY 3: Low-Carb Day

DAY 4: High-Carb Day (includes a reward meal)

DAY 5: Low-Carb Day

DAY 6: High-Carb Day

DAY 7: Low-Carb Day

Cycle Option #2 – Activate Hot Cycle

The Activate Hot Cycle is slightly more challenging, because the Moderate Cycle has less high-carb days and a no-carb day. Don't worry, it still has a couple high-carb days and a reward meal.

As I said, adjust the cycle days to the days of the week where you will thrive best. It might be wise to have your high-carb (reward meal) day on a weekend.

CYCLE PROTOCOL:

DAY 1: High-Carb Day

DAY 2: Low-Carb Day

DAY 3: Low-Carb Day

DAY 4: High-Carb Day (includes a reward meal)

DAY 5: Low-Carb Day

DAY 6: Medium-Carb Day

DAY 7: No-Carb Day

Cycle Option #3 – The Accelerated Inferno Cycle

The Accelerated Inferno Cycle takes carb cycling to the next level for sure. This carb cycle is the most challenging of the three. Make sure you are ready, I mean mentally prepared for a challenge. During this cycle, you will quickly see what you're made of.

With two no-carb days in this cycle, you will burn fat like crazy. You will likely experience a dip in your energy levels, it is what it is so plan accordingly (see tips below) Get your most important stuff done on your high-carb days, trust me, haha—because on the high-carb days, your energy levels will be at their peak.

Do not start here, please. If you've never done a carb cycling plan before, start with the first two cycles.

CYCLE PROTOCOL:

DAY 1: High-Carb Day

DAY 2: Low-Carb Day

DAY 3: No-Carb Day

DAY 4: High-Carb Day (includes a reward meal)

DAY 5: No-Carb Day

DAY 6: Low-Carb Day

DAY 7: Medium-Carb Day

In the next section, you'll learn portion sizes as well as the methodology for each type of day. Pay very close attention so you know what you can and cannot do in order to see the greatest results on your new diet.

Portioning Your Meals

One of the most important aspects of successfully losing weight is regulating your portions. In this section, I will teach you how to portion out all five meals for each type of carb day. Over the years, we have become very accustomed to large portion sizes without really thinking about how this affects our ability to maintain a healthy weight. With the easy measuring tools I am about to teach you, you will soon be able to create just the right portions at each meal for your body.

These portion sizes have been shown to be a very good and accurate measure for most people (there's always an exception to the rule). You will use your hand to measure portions, and since your hand is proportionate to the size of your frame, it's a great way to measure consumption.

MEASURING YOUR PORTIONS	
PROTEINS [meat, poultry, or seafood]	1 serving of protein [meat, poultry, or seafood] should be equal to the size of the palm of your hand or a little bigger.
CARBOHYDRATES	Your portion of carbohydrates [1 serving] should be the size of your clenched fist.
VEGETABLES	Your portion of veggies is the size of 2 clenched fists. Remember veggies can be eaten freely on the Sweet Potato Diet.
FATS	Size of your thumb joint to the tip, or a little more.
FLAVORINGS	If your flavorings are calorie-free, feel free to season to your liking. There are many seasonings that have little or no calories. At my house, we use Flavor God. If your seasonings are calorically dense, please use sparingly or not at all.

Building a High-Carb, Medium-Carb, Low-Carb, or No-Carb Meal

HIGH CARB MEAL	• **PROTEIN (MEAT, POULTRY, OR SEAFOOD):** 1 portion the size of the palm of your hand or a little bit more. • **CARBOHYDRATES:** 2 portions the size of 2 clenched fists. • **VEGETABLES:** 1 portion the size of your clenched fist or more. • **FATS:** 1 portion the size of your thumb joint to the tip.
MEDIUM CARB MEAL	• **PROTEIN (MEAT, POULTRY, OR SEAFOOD):** 1 portion the size of the palm of your hand or a little bit more. • **CARBOHYDRATES:** 1 portion the size of one clenched fist. • **VEGETABLES:** 2 portions the size of two clenched fists or more. • **FATS:** 1 portion the size of your thumb joint to the tip.
LOW CARB MEAL	• **PROTEIN (MEAT, POULTRY, OR SEAFOOD):** 1 portion the size of the palm of your hand. • **CARBOHYDRATES:** ½ portion the size of half of your fist. • **VEGETABLES:** 2 portions the size of two clenched fists or more. • **FATS:** 2–3 portions the size of your thumb joint to the tip.
NO CARB MEAL	• **PROTEIN (MEAT, POULTRY, OR SEAFOOD):** 1 portion the size of the palm of your hand. You could even double protein here. • **CARBOHYDRATES:** 0 portions. There are no sweet potatoes on these days. • **VEGETABLES:** 2 portions the size of two clenched fists or more. • **FATS:** 2–3 portions the size of your thumb joint to the tip.

That's it. You'll never have to wonder about proper portion sizes again. Just use your hands as your guide, and begin reaping the rewards of the Sweet Potato Diet almost instantly. Are you ready for some of my best carb-cycling tips? These tips continue to save me every week, and without them my family couldn't put up with me on no-carb days, haha!

LOW- AND NO-CARB DAY TIPS

There's no question these will be your most difficult days, especially initially as your body learns how to function on less fuel. Here are some of my best tips, and if you follow me on Snapchat, these are the tips you'll see me use on my low- and no-carb days.

1. Sip BCAAs throughout your low and no-carb days. These are especially important on these days for two reasons; first because BCAAs ward off hunger, and secondly, because they have been shown to preserve lean muscle tissue. And, since you are in a catabolic state on these days, the preservation of muscle becomes even more critical. I use my own brand for numerous reasons, most importantly there's no sucrose, nothing artificial, no dyes, and no fillers—not to mention they taste like an orange dreamsicle. You can learn more by visiting www.morellifit.com/bcaas.

2. Drink even more water. This along with your BCAAs will keep hunger in check.

3. Stock up on veggies, in fact, slice up some veggie sticks so you have them available. You will get hungry and since these are free carbs you can munch away.

4. Pre-make some extra protein. In the event you get hungry and the veggies don't satisfy your hunger, grab some lean protein.

5. If the veggies and the protein don't do it, you can slightly increase fats. I suggest sticking with avocado here though.

6. Stay busy! I mean it. We often get hungry because we are bored. When you stay, busy your mind stays occupied. How often do you get lost in what you're doing, look up and realize three hours have gone by since you last ate. Get into this flow, especially on your low and no-carb days.

These six things will undoubtedly make your hardest days become manageable, setting you up for major success on this diet. I invite you to implement all six of them on your low- and no-carb days. Remember, I've gone before you. I know exactly what it takes to thrive on this diet.

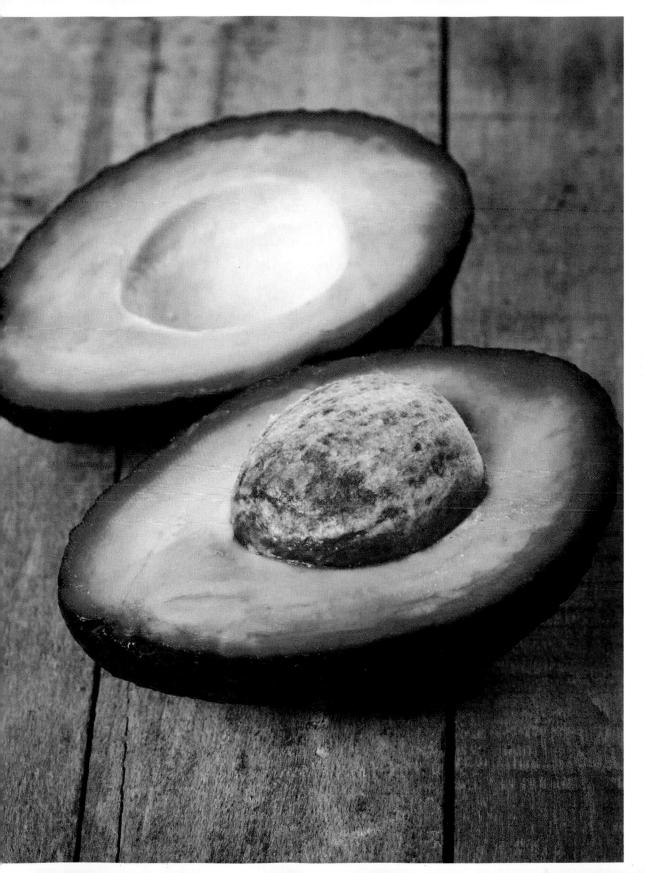

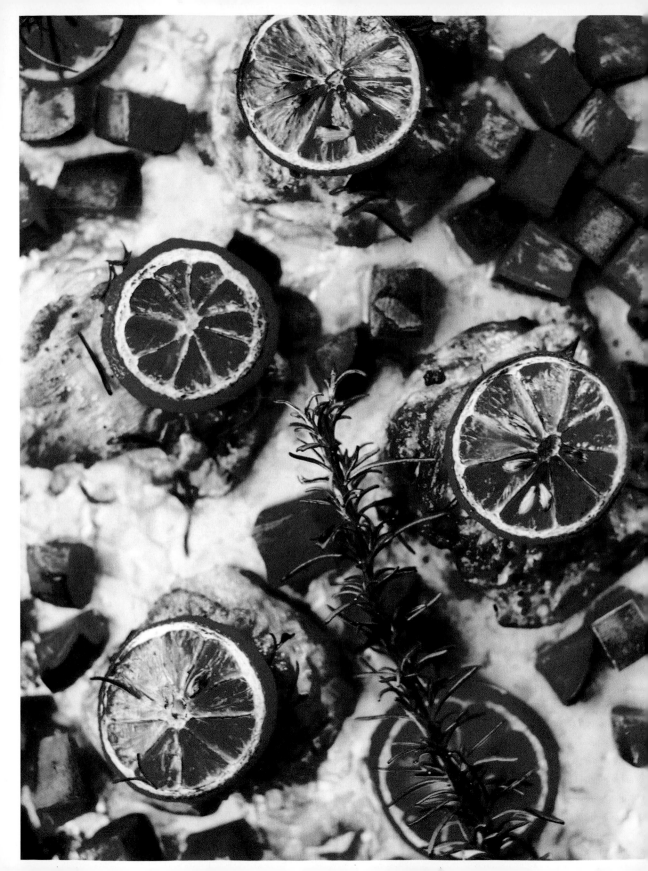

CHAPTER 7:

How to Track Results and Read the Signs

invite you to track your progress. It's something I wish I would have done from the very start three years ago when it all began for me. You can't improve what you don't measure, and there are several measures we will use on the Sweet Potato Diet. With that in mind, it's very important not to get fixated on the scale. Remember, my diet is designed to help you burn fat while preserving lean muscle tissue. To give you an example; I weigh more today than I did three years ago and I was 24 plus percent body fat, now I live at around eight. The scale doesn't take into account muscle vs fat mass ratio, it doesn't measure water weight either, and so on this diet I ask you to take it with a grain a salt.

Let me break it down really quick for you. Your weight will fluctuate. In the beginning of the book if you remember, your body can fluctuate 5 or so pounds on any given day. This is on its own as a result of an array of factors, to name a few, water and food consumption and of course hormones play a huge role, as well.

In the past, I have told my clients to stay off the scale for this reason and it always works in their favor. For those that have heads like rocks, it's been a thorn in their side. You see, when you're fixated on a number, your mind runs, stress and anxiety plague you making it even harder to drop body fat. I have only worked with a couple hundred thousand people, what do I know? That was a joke! Sorry I had to! Just listen to me, damn it!

Stay away from the scale in the beginning. I mean it. Do not weigh yourself for the first 30 days, and then after 30 days, no more than every two weeks max. Here are some much better tools to use instead.

CLOTHING AND INCHES—Taking measurements is a good indicator; arms, waist, hips, and thighs are all great ways to track progress. My personal favorite is being aware of how my clothes fit and look on me. There's nothing like feeling good in a nice outfit. Set goals and treat yourself.

ENERGY LEVELS—While this one isn't too sexy, it's a good one and it's almost always overlooked. Pay attention to your energy levels, clarity, and focus. It's very common that people experience much better energy throughout the day on the Sweet Potato Diet. And, if you decide to workout (which I strongly encourage) you will increase stamina and energy throughout your day tenfold. This is a sign to look out for and a marker that you are making progress.

APPETITE AND CRAVINGS—Your appetite and cravings will also begin to shift. As your body and palate adjust to healthier whole foods, your cravings for simple carbohydrates and sugars will diminish over time. You will become much more sensitive to and aware of the very "sweet" and the very "salty" tastes. These are all great indicators of great progress toward healthier, more vibrant living.

MOOD—This is potentially my favorite, because prior to my transformation a was a moody little bastard. That has since changed. Not to mention with a combination of healthy nutrition and supplementation (more on supplementation later). I was able to kick my anti-depression meds. You can expect to see less mood swings, it's actually quite common.

How Can I Create Enough Time for Meal Prep?

Meal prep is a major struggle for most people as they transition away from convenience and fast food to a healthier way of eating. Let me be blunt. If you don't make time for your wellness, you will make time for your illness. My good friend and expert nutritionist Brian Johnson says this all the time, and he's right!

After working with hundreds of thousands of clients, there's one thing I have learned, in order to be successful you must stay prepared. Here are the top tips from those in my private Facebook group:

- Set aside 2-3 hours each Sunday (or whatever day works for your schedule) to prepare the entire week's meals;
- Cook dinner every night and make enough extra to take with you the next day;
- Pay to have someone else prep for you. I am serious. It all depends on what the opportunity costs is for your time. You can find someone online for about $15/hr. Is it worth it for you to pay someone $60 or so per week to do it for you? You'll have to decide. We have someone come twice per week. It wasn't always like that, but now my time is more valuable than what I could pay someone to prep for me, so I elect to do it that way.

Once you've decided on how you will approach food prep, here are some action items that helped me:

- Review your upcoming schedule. What do you need, when will you be busy, when will you be out and about? What challenges might you face? You can never be too prepared.
- Create your menu for at least the next two to three days. Choose delicious meals and recipes from the Sweet Potato Diet meal planner, recipe guide, and grocery list.
- Build a grocery list from your menu. The Sweet Potato Diet meal planner makes this a cinch. All you have to do is choose your meals from the planner, then buy the necessary ingredients, all of which are approved foods on the Sweet Potato Diet.

Take a trip to your grocery store and get everything you need, preferably for the entire week all in one trip.

Decide when the best time to prep is. Schedule it. If you can schedule the shopping and the prep all in the same afternoon, I suggest doing that. Sunday was always a good day for me.

Cravings: How to Easily Curb Them

Cravings can be one of your worst enemies. And trust me, I love sweets and carbs just like you. So here's a few things that tend to help when the cravings strike.

> **WATER**—Slam a glass of water. The more water you drink the better off you will be. It's essential, anyways, silly. So drink it. You know what? Have a glass right now as you're reading the chapter. There's your reminder for today. I carry a big jug around with me everywhere I go, and yes, I even bring it into restaurants with me. It keeps me on track.

> **GRAB A MINT**—After slamming a glass of water, I usually pop a mint, and since craving usually strike me at night, I quickly take my ass to bed. *LOL*. Seriously though, I do.

> **DARK CHOCOLATE CHIPS**—If I still need something, I reach for a stash of dark chocolate chips (60% cocoa or better). Ten or so little chips usually does the trick and they won't derail you if you stop at ten.

> **SWEET POTATOES**—Prepare one of the Sweet Potato Desserts or throw some cinnamon on them. This always works for me, too.

A couple more things to consider with regard to cravings.

FIBER AND FATS

Fiber provides satiety and helps you to feel full for longer. It also slows the release of glucose into your bloodstream, which helps with fat loss. Finally, fiber slows down digestion, so it will take longer for you to feel hungry after meals. This is a huge benefit of sweet potatoes.

The same thing with fats. They keep you fuller longer. As mentioned previously, this is especially important on low- and no-carb days. Make sure you stick to the plan, eat your healthy fats.

When you combine all of the above tools and eat according to plan (fats and fiber) it's very hard to get derailed by a craving. They will happen. It's inevitable. Fight them with the tools above. Think about your health and your new physique.

SUPER CARB CYCLING TROUBLESHOOTING

In order for the Sweet Potato Diet to work, you must follow the blueprint as I have laid it out. Remember in the beginning I told you I removed all of the fluff? I left only the parts that are 100% necessary for success and I took everything else out.

This is the section to use if you have trouble getting started or if you ever hit a plateau. We can sort it out quickly, give you a swift kick in the butt (because that's likely what you need), and get you back on the road to success. I'm right here with you—my promise!

HOW IMPORTANT IS THE EATING SCHEDULE?

In order for the diet to work, it's critical that you eat five meals daily at approximately three-hour intervals. Does that mean there won't be days where you only get four in? No. It means do your best to get five in as much as possible. This is what your body needs to become a fat-burning machine. Please refer back to the section on meal frequency if need be.

HOW BAD IS IT IF I CHEAT?

Bad! Cheaters never win. It's true here, too. There's built-in reward meals every week, sweet potato desserts you can substitute in, and I just said you could have ten dark chocolate chips if you absolutely need to in order to fight off a craving late at night. But that's it!

No matter how hard you work, if you take in more calories than your body burns over the course of the diet, you will not lose weight—period.

WHAT HAPPENS IF I DON'T WANT TO EAT THIS MUCH?

Eating too little is also detrimental to your success. If you are not feeding your body adequately, it will adjust its level of metabolism (by slowing it down) to conserve energy, and will begin to store fat for the future. You have to eat enough calories to "feed the burn" and encourage your body to work more efficiently.

WHAT IF I DON'T EXERCISE?

What if you die early? I don't know. Later in the book, there's a short chapter on exercise. Can you give me 5 minutes a day first thing in the morning? You picked up this book for a reason. Give it 30 days and then decide if it's been worth it. Deal?

I'M NOT SEEING RESULTS?

First of all, are you not seeing any results or just not seeing them as fast as you'd like? There's a big difference. Everyone is different and experiences success at a different rate. Here are a few hacks I've worked up over the years, please make the following adjustments and make sure to follow the plan 100%.

1. Work all of your portions of carbohydrates for the day either into the first three meals, or split all of your allotted carbs into three and consume them for breakfast, before training, and right after you're done training.

2. Eat the remaining portions of proteins, fats, and veggies in the rest of the meals for the day. You will still be eating all of your portions for the day, you'll just be eating all the carbs early on in the day.

3. Replace one of your low-carb days with a no-carb day. Preferably the one after your high-carb day.

4. Eliminate your reward meal for the next two weeks. Hey how bad do you want it? That's what I thought.

5. Add 10 minutes of exercise to your daily regimen.

Feel free to give one of these a go or all of them at once. The choice is yours. You will win trust me, stay the course. These changes should help stimulate fat loss. And if for whatever reason they don't? I'm going to share a big secret: my "Plateau Breaker."

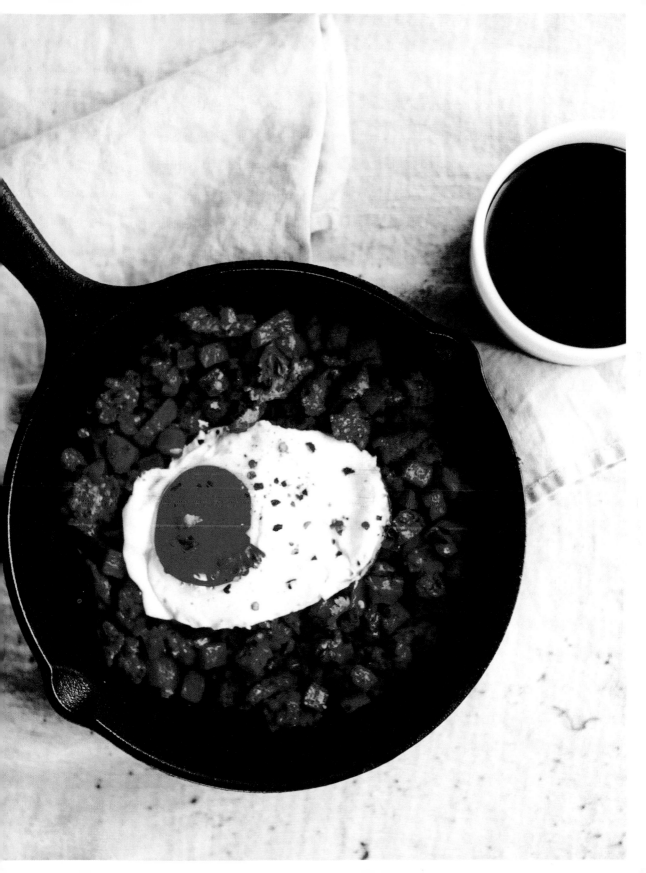

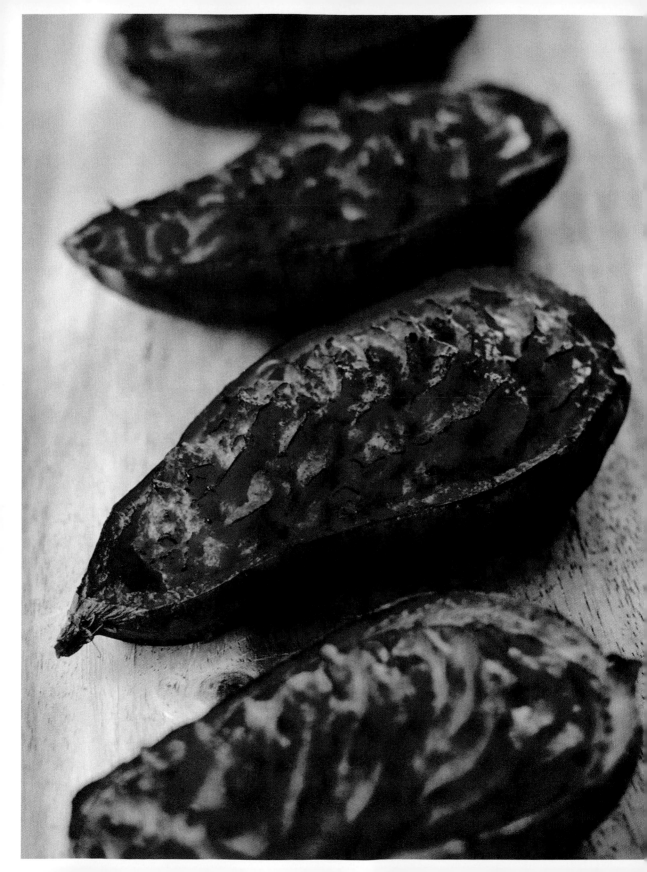

CHAPTER 8:

Busting Out the Big Guns:
The Plateau Breaker

How Did I Hit a Plateau?

So here's the reality, some people react quickly to the carb cycles and can keep losing for a long time. Others lose at first but then plateau. Carb cycling is the most effective way to offset your metabolism's ability to adapt. But at some point, it may eventually adapt to carb cycling. I'm just being honest. (I don't want to mislead you—I'm here to provide solutions, not false promises.)

If your fat loss stalls or stops, it means your highly intelligent body has learned the pattern and is adapting to conserve as much energy (fat) as possible.

Your body may reach this stage during your journey on the Sweet Potato Diet. DO NOT quit, there's solutions out there for everything. In fact, I enjoy a good challenge!

If your body adapts, turn the tables with my Plateau Breaker.

The Plateau Breaker is a great tool to use, if necessary. Once implemented, your body is forced to reset and boost its metabolism.

What Is the Plateau Breaker?

On other weight loss programs, the dieter's plateau is more often than not the straw that breaks the camel's back. Not with the Sweet Potato Diet. In fact, the antidote is here. Because I have helped so many achieve success, there isn't much I haven't seen or have had to overcome for clients. This is no different. It happens, and we deal with it.

So your metabolism has figured out our carb cycle and you've stopped losing fat. That just means we need to shock your body yet again with a new eating pattern, something it hasn't seen before. This more often than not restarts your metabolism, so you can break through and begin shedding fat again.

By using the Plateau Breaker, you won't get stuck on the dieter's plateau—you'll break right through it and get back to torching fat. All you need to do is to "periodize" your weekly nutrition: the single most effective way to keep your body from figuring out what you're trying to do.

To do this, take seven high-carbohydrate days in a row. This revs your metabolism, fills your body with nutritious food, and primes you to lose weight again. I know hearing this may scare you a bit, but it works. During this week, you should not have any reward meals. Stick to the cycle and make sure sweet potatoes are your only carbohydrate.

Your body will notice you're not having any low-carb days that week, and it will relax, assuming there's no reason to conserve. You'll resume burning tons of calories and fat. Once your metabolism pumps up in your *breakthrough* week, you throw it a curveball by dropping back into a 7-day carb cycle the very next week.

No matter how adaptive your system is, it can't adjust in time, and fat loss is inevitable. The Plateau Breaker clears the slate to help get your body back on track.

How to Break Through Your Plateau

Clients do come to me from time to time with challenges. After we have helped over 200,000 people directly, and who knows how many more through social media, it's bound to happen. It's usually because they have hit a plateau or are not losing fat at the rate they would like.

Contradictory to what the doctors and most of the world would say, when they increase their daily calorie intake, their fat loss actually picks up steam. I know it sounds crazy, I was on the fence when I learned this methodology, too, but it has worked again and again, and it will work for you. You won't gain fat, even though you're eating more. Maybe some water weight, but not fat.

Your intuitive response to a dieter's plateau will probably be to eat less and exercise more. DON'T DO IT. You'll just become more firmly stuck where you are. What you need is a *breakthrough*.

So, how do you implement the Plateau Breaker and guarantee that your body will keep losing fat? It's unbelievably simple.

- 3 weeks of the 7-day carb cycle
- 1 week of the breakthrough cycle

Depending on your body, your weight may remain the same during this week, or you may lose a significant amount of weight. Don't panic if you gain a little weight. It's solely due to water retention, and the water will flush as you return to your carb cycles. If you level off instead of losing, don't worry. When you resume carb cycling, you'll be cruising at high speed again.

So, don't vary the protocol. Stay the course.

That's the secret to consistent and sustainable fat loss. No more mystery to the dieter's plateau. Now, YOU are in control.

GUIDELINES FOR THE BREAKTHROUGH CYCLE:

- For 1 week, every day is a high-carb day.
- Eat 5 meals every day.
- Choose from the list of approved foods.
- Measure the right portion sizes for YOU.
- At all five of your daily meals, include your correct portion of carbs, proteins, fats, and veggies.
- Eat within 30 to 60 minutes of waking and every three hours thereafter.
- Drink half of your body weight in ounces of water each day, absolute minimum.

PART 3:
THE RECIPES

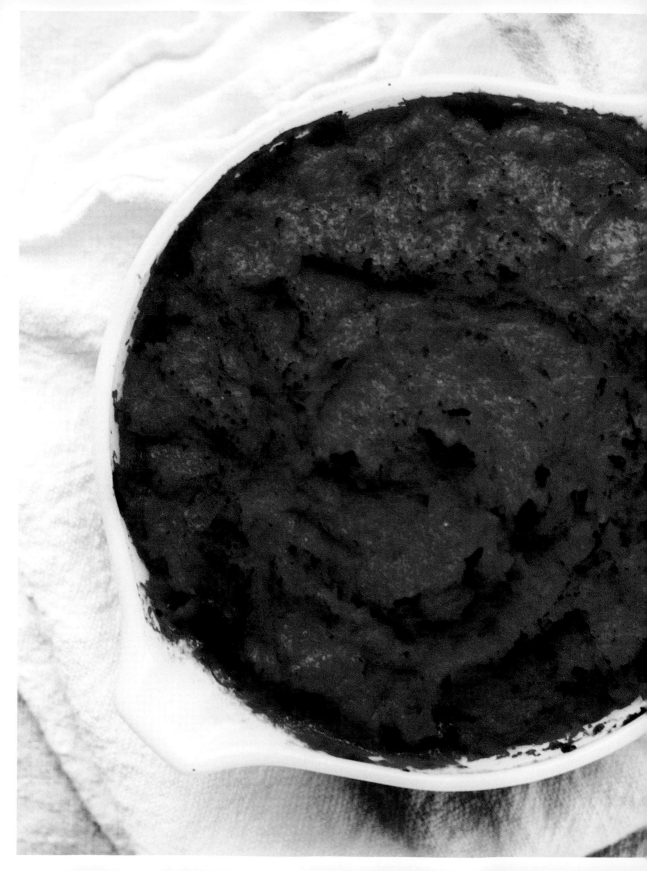

CHAPTER 9:

The Sweet Potato Diet Success Tips—Adopting the Lifestyle of Permanent Fat Loss

Using the Recipes in Your Carb Cycle

These are all delicious and bring a wide variety of flavors and fun into all of your meals. The best way to measure these recipes into your meal plan is to use the guidelines for measuring carbohydrate portions. The fist portion sizing works for the recipes as well. We know some have more or less sweet potato in them, but the key is not to stress, because the sweet potato is a power carb and these recipes are super clean. So, in recipes a little more or less is OK. Enjoy them!

All of the recipes in the Sweet Potato Diet are carb heavy and should be first considered carbohydrate portions when working them into your carb cycles, even though they likely contain other macros. For the recipes that are higher in protein, you can factor it in if you'd like. But remember, if you go back and take a look at the section on portioning, you'll see where I mention more protein throughout the day won't hinder your progress and is ok. If a recipe contains lots of healthy fats, please consider them and make adjustments during the day to support the additional fats. A good rule of thumb, since you'll utilize the recipes mostly on high- and medium-carb days, is if a recipe contains fat, that should be your only fat intake. Don't add it to any of your other meals throughout the day. This will keep you in the safe zone.

Success Tips

You've heard me talk about all of my amazing clients, hundreds of thousands in fact. You know why that is so great for you? Because through all of their success and failures, we have learned what works and what doesn't and have compiled a list of tips that will help you create success on your journey.

I encourage you to really absorb these tips, maybe even print them out and put them somewhere you'll see them every day (in your wallet, in your training diary, or on your refrigerator) and turn to them if you're ever in doubt...

- Use the Sweet Potato Diet grocery/food lists, meal planner, and recipes.
- Schedule time(s) for grocery shopping, meal prep, and cooking.
- Select delicious recipes from the Sweet Potato Diet recipe guide.
- Enjoy only approved foods from the Sweet Potato Diet approved foods and grocery list.
- Be sure to eat all your carbs when your cycle calls for them.
- Your most active days should be scheduled on your high carb days whenever possible.
- On your low- or no-carb days, keep exercise short.
- Never skip breakfast.
- Always eat protein with every meal.
- Don't eat processed carbs, or any junk for that matter.
- Drink plenty of water each day (half your body weight; 200 lbs = 100 oz water min).
- Enjoy non-starchy veggies, eat them as freely as you'd like, especially on your low- and no-carb days.
- Stay active (workouts later in the book).
- Weigh yourself only every two weeks (same time, preferably upon awaking, and if you can, on the same day of the carb cycle).
- Be patient and stay the course.
- Don't pay attention to the negative people.

Lifestyle of Permanent Weight Management

After you've reached your goal weight, then what?

You get to decide. One thing I can promise you is there's very little chance of rebound as long as you don't do anything crazy. You have had carbs, reward meals, and the occasional sweet treat, that's the beauty of the Sweet Potato Diet. You haven't been deprived, which means the yo-yo breaks and stops here.

Congratulations! Can you see yourself at the finish line? In those jeans? Who are you with? What are people saying?

You've finally made it. You've achieved your goal, and you've worked your ass off—lots of hard work, the discipline to stay the course, and the determination to finish what you started!

I am so damn proud of you!

Take the time to appreciate both the little and the big wins on your journey and to realize how awesome your achievement is. Most of the world stays stuck, becomes a statistic, but you made it out! Now you are likely experiencing things you thought might never be possible:

- Playing with your kids without getting winded
- Receiving compliments from strangers
- Feeling the elation of success and accomplishment
- Feeling in control
- Making your health the priority it deserves
- Exercising daily
- Wearing a two-piece swimsuit, sleeveless dress, or form-fitting clothes
- Maybe you've decided to participate in a fitness event
- Waking up every day feeling energized

Take a moment to make a list of all of the things you are grateful for. It doesn't matter whether you've achieved your goals or not, it's only a matter of time before you do. We all have things we can be grateful for.

The simpler they are, the better. Some of mine include; heath, clean running water, my family, and the ability to eat really healthy food every day.

How to Maintain Success for Life

Ah, yes! Success for life, something we all strive for. Here's a few principles that I follow, whether I am carb cycling or not. They have had huge positive implications on my overall well-being, and I know they will do the same for you. These are little guidelines you can pass along to your family, too.

EAT BREAKFAST. I truly believe that breakfast is the most important meal of the day. When you wake up, it's been somewhere between 8 and 15 hours since your last meal. Your body needs nourishment and energy. By eating breakfast within an hour of waking, you jump-start your body's metabolism and get it primed for burning fat throughout the day. Various studies have shown that people who skip breakfast have a tendency to overeat at the next meal (because they're hungry). Eat a balanced, nutritious breakfast, and start your day right.

EAT OFTEN. You have learned about your body's metabolism. Eating smaller meals often benefits you in several ways. It keeps your digestive system continually active and burning energy. Eating smaller meals at more frequent intervals keeps you from getting hungry, and your body will continually feel satisfied, you won't have cravings, and you'll avoid the temptation to overeat on junk.

EAT BALANCED MEALS. Stick to lean meats, a little bit of fruit, sweet potatoes, lots of veggies, and some nuts and seeds, and you will thrive. This ensures your body will convert the majority of calories that you eat into usable energy, not stored fat. Good nourishment is good for your body, mind, and soul.

CONTROL YOUR PORTIONS. Don't starve yourself, deprive yourself a variety of foods, or skip meals in an attempt to drop fat, ever. Simply remember to control your meal portions and stay on the right track for maintaining your ideal body weight. Yes, it's hard to think about portion control in a world where everything seems super-sized. Do your best, nothing more and nothing less.

TRAIN YOUR BODY TO BE SATISFIED WITH LESS FOOD. When you eat smaller portions and enjoy your food at a leisurely pace, your brain has time to recognize what you're eating. You'll feel satisfied. If you rush through a meal, your brain doesn't have time to catch up. By the time it does, maybe you've already overeaten.

BALANCE BLOOD GLUCOSE LEVELS. Balanced glucose and insulin levels are extremely important to maintaining a healthy, fat-burning metabolism. When you eat, your body turns the food you eat into glucose (sugar), which it uses as energy or stores as fat. Insulin is produced by your pancreas to shuttle the glucose into your cells. But when you eat large meal portions, your blood sugar levels rise sharply. Your pancreas releases too much insulin which then leads to low blood sugar. Your brain then thinks you don't have enough glucose which triggers feelings of hunger (often for sugar). And so a vicious cycle of high and low blood sugar ensues. By controlling meal portions, you help your body maintain stable glucose and insulin levels, which in turn leads to less cravings.

DRINK PLENTY OF WATER. Your body is up to 60% water and needs it to function properly. Three-fourths of the water inside your body is inside your body's cells. In addition to your cells, your body needs water to digest food properly, regulate its temperature, eliminate waste, and more. Having adequate water intake helps your body function at its best and plays a huge role in weight management.

MOVE. Your body was designed to move. Regular physical activity helps you feel better, mentally and physically. It helps burn sufficient amounts of energy so that your body doesn't store fat. But physical activity also helps you to build and maintain muscle tissue which creates a need for more energy. Finally, physical activity reduces your risk of weight-related diseases, such as type 2 diabetes, cancer, and high blood pressure. It also helps you to sleep better and helps your mood. So move!

SLEEP. The importance of sleep cannot be stressed enough. Sleep is just as important as training and nutrition. You simply can't catch up on sleep. If you have to choose between sleep and training, go with sleep. Why? Because you can't get the desired effects from training without adequate sleep. Lack of sleep or a disruption in your circadian rhythm will increase the stress hormone cortisol. Add intense training on top of poor sleep and you have one big mess. If you're feeling drained from a bad night's sleep, listen to your body. Maybe do some mobility work, go for a walk outside, or do some light aerobic cardio. But do not put your body through an intense session if you're exhausted from bad night's rest. PS: It's OK to nap. I am not talking about 3-hour naps, but just enough in the middle of the day to restore your mind. There are days when instead of reaching for more coffee I just allow my body to run the show, and that means closing my eyes for 20–30 minutes. Sometimes I fall asleep, many times I don't, but I always feel restored and ready for the next project.

These are the fundamental habits that have helped me stay focused and consistent with my health, and I invite you to join me and the many others who have made these habits rituals in their lives and are reaping the major benefits they have to offer. You deserve to look and feel your best.

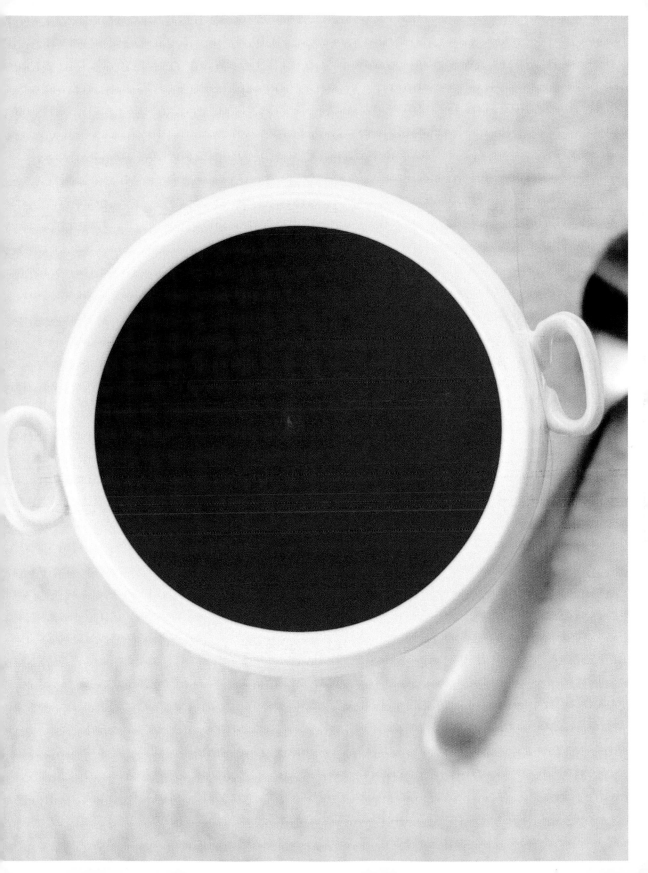

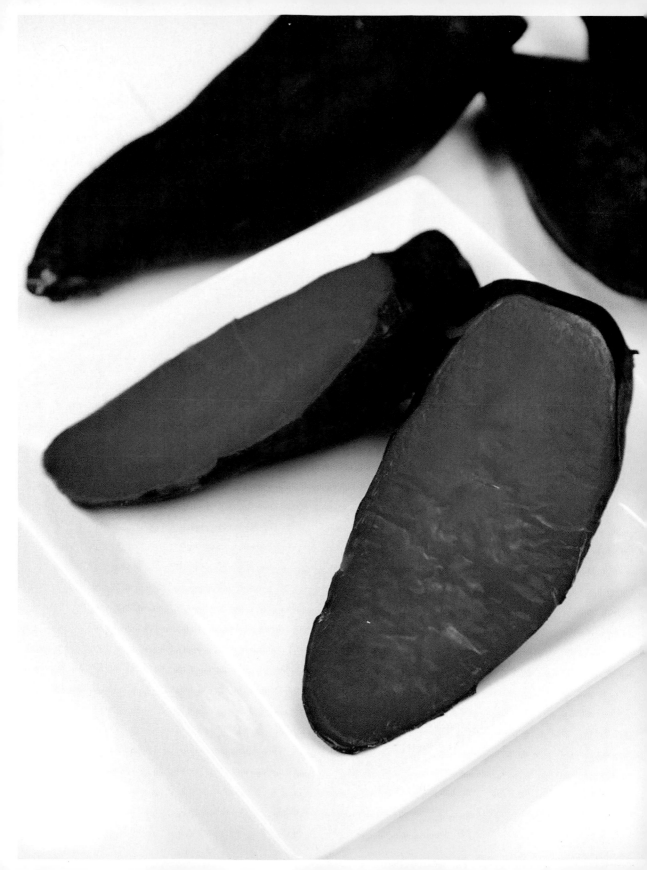

CHAPTER 10:

Sweet Potato Prep, Approved Foods, and the Grocery Guide

What Are the Best Types of Sweet Potatoes?

There are many different types of sweet potatoes, and they come in a wide variety of colors, textures, and flavors. The flesh in particular can range from your traditional white and orange to a vivid purple. The color of the sweet potato actually correlates with the potato's nutritional content, so the more intense the color, the more nutritional value it has.

[ORANGE SWEET POTATO] ORANGE/RED SKIN AND ORANGE FLESH: These are the sweet potatoes that most people think of when you mention the word sweet potato; they have become popular in the American diet. In the US, this sweet potato is commonly labeled as a yam, although traditionally, the two are nothing alike and are from two different botanical families. The traditional yam is not something you would find in your local supermarket, but rather something you would pick up from a specialty grocery store. The orange sweet potato is known for its soft, sweet orange flesh and is now a staple at the Thanksgiving dinner table.

There are many individual types of orange sweet potatoes, but the most popular type found in the United States is called the Beauregard and is grown in Louisiana.

(JAPANESE SWEET POTATO) PURPLE SKIN AND BUTTER-COLORED FLESH:
The Japanese sweet potato is a common type of sweet potato used in Japan and can also be found at some specialty stores. These sweet potatoes are known for being denser and sweeter than the traditional orange sweet potato. They were even promoted as being the top superfood of 2010 by Dr. Oz.

(OKINAWAN SWEET POTATO) GRAY OR TAN SKIN AND PURPLE FLESH: The Okinawan sweet potato is known for its health benefits and for being high in antioxidants, which is actually what gives this potato its vibrant purple flesh. This sweet potato, which is native to the US, is popular in Japan and Hawaii and has a delicate, creamy texture that is slightly sweet.

(WHITE SWEET POTATO) PALE YELLOW SKIN AND BUTTER-COLORED FLESH:
The white sweet potato is drier and less sweet than the orange sweet potato, but still a popular sweet potato in the United States. This milder sweet potato is good for someone who is looking for a less intense flavor from their sweet potato.

Any of the above work just fine. I actually love the white sweet potatoes; they are my favorite of them all. If you've never had them, I strongly suggest the next time you're at the store picking up a few. If you thought the orange sweet potatoes were good, wait until you give the white ones a go. Yum!

How Do I Know I Am Not Buying Yams?

The most common sweet potato used in the American diet is the bright orange one. When looking at sweet potatoes, which may often times be labeled as a yam (at least in the US), you should still know the difference, only to ensure you're getting a sweet potato and not a yam. Chances are, the yam will be a sweet potato, as real yams aren't as common in the United States.

A real yam is a starchy African root with the outside being brown, rough, and scaly with a whiter flesh, while the orange sweet potato has orange or red skin with orange flesh. The reason that the orange sweet potato is often called a yam is because when it was being introduced to the American market, producers and shippers wanted the sweet potato to stand out and not be confused with the more traditional potato. This is where the confusion arose. Sellers continue to sell them as yams for the simple reason that people like to buy them that way, too.

When you go to buy sweet potatoes, there are a few things you should be on the lookout for:

- Look for the sweet potatoes that have smooth skin, are free of blemishes, and are small to medium sized. In fact, picking ones that are the size of your closed fist is the easiest way to pick potatoes that are portioned for you. Might as well kill two birds with one stone. Buying them close to the size you need for your meals just makes it easier for you during prep.
- Make sure that the sweet potato is clean, firm, and free of any mold.
- Always avoid sweet potatoes that have soft spots, blemishes, or mold. This will change the taste of the sweet potato, even if you cut that part off. When one part of the sweet potato begins to mold, the flavor can actually spread throughout the entire potato.

You know I probably should have asked in the beginning of the book: Do you say PO-TATE-OH or PA-*TAH-TOH? Lol.*

Just curious. Did you know the best tasting sweet potatoes are found during the fall and winter months? It's during this time when they are naturally in season.

How Do I Store and Keep My Sweet Potatoes Fresh?

Once you get your sweet potatoes home, you should store them until you are ready to cook.

Don't put them in the refrigerator. I have seen this countless times. Believe it or not, refrigeration can make them starchy, as the natural sugars turn to starch. Not to mention, they can become hard in the center and tougher to cook, sometimes not softening even after they've been cooked.

So, store your sweet potatoes in a cool, dry place, around 55–65° F. They should last a couple of weeks if stored properly. Good places to store them are in dark corners of your pantry or in a cupboard that closes to keep out the light.

While you should avoid the refrigerator, it is possible to store your sweet potatoes in the freezer, if done properly. If you decide to do this, cook your sweet potatoes first, allow them to cool completely, and then place them in an airtight freezer bag. Sweet potatoes can keep in the freezer for up to 6 months. This is a great way to speed up food prep for those who are super busy. I like to cut them into fours, bake them, and then store them this way. Pull them out, heat them up, add some pink Himalayan salt and you've got sweet potato bars—great for on-the-go.

What's The Easiest Way to Prep Sweet Potatoes?

There are tons ways to prep your sweet potatoes and each brings some different flavors. When you're cooking your sweet potatoes, it is best to leave the skin on (I actually eat the skin), unless the preparation calls for you to peel it, as the skin of the sweet potato has almost ten times as much antioxidant power as the flesh. The nutritional value can fluctuate a bit based on prep. Learn to enjoy the skin, I actually love it!

When preparing your sweet potato, always use a stainless steel knife to chop and cut to avoid changing the color of the sweet potato.

> **BAKING:** Baking your sweet potato is a popular option and can be really tasty as it breaks down the natural sugars, allowing it to caramelize as it cooks. Begin by preheating your oven to 400° F. Poke your sweet potato with a fork so that there are little holes all over it. Once your oven is heated, bake your sweet potato for 45–60 minutes, depending on the sweet potato's size and the power of your oven. You'll know it's ready when you can easily puncture it with a knife. The outside should be crispy and the inside nice and soft. When you slice the potato open, the inside of the skin should be black, charred from the caramelized sugars. If you are meal prepping and want to save your potato for later, you can store it in the refrigerator or freezer by sticking it in an airtight freezer bag after letting it cool down to room temperature.

> **BOILING:** Boiling your sweet potato can be a great way to retain the antioxidant power and is also a simple, quick preparation. Because the skin of the sweet potato is so nutritious, you will want to boil the sweet potato whole rather than cutting it into smaller pieces or peeling it. Fill your pot

with enough water to cover your potato (usually about half full) and bring to a boil. Place your whole sweet potato in the water and allow it to cook for about 20-30 minutes, or until the potato is tender enough to be pierced with a knife. Remove your sweet potato and proceed to peel it once it has cooled. You can then either slice it up and serve or mash it for a yummy alternative to traditional mashed potatoes.

GRILLING: Sweet potatoes make a great side when you are cooking outside on the grill in the summertime. Preheat your grill on high. Once the grill is heated, slice your sweet potatoes in half and place skin side down. Close the grill and let them cook for 30 minutes or until your liking.

MICROWAVING: Microwaving your sweet potato can be a good option when you don't have a lot of time on your hands, and although you will be missing out on the caramelization of the sugars in the sweet potato, this can still be a tasty alternative to baking. Using a fork, poke holes all over your sweet potato and microwave it on high for 4–5 minutes. Turn over and repeat. Once done, the sweet potato should be soft enough to easily pierce with a knife. I don't use the microwave much these days, and if at all possible do your best to avoid it. It's just not the best way to cook or warm up food.

SAUTÉING: Peel your sweet potato and cut it into either slices, strips, or cubes. Using a nonstick pan, heat oil (preferably coconut) on medium-low heat. Add in the pieces of sweet potato and sauté until your liking. This is a quick way to bring out the natural sweetness of the sweet potato. By cutting your sweet potato into 'fries,' this is can also be a healthier alternative to traditional French fries.

STEAMING: You can either steam your sweet potato whole or cut it into half-inch slices and steam them that way, both unpeeled. Fill your steamer so that there is 2–3 inches of water at the bottom. Once the steam builds up, add your sweet potato and let cook. Sliced sweet potato should take 7–10 minutes, while a whole sweet potato cooks for 30 minutes, or until it is soft enough to easily pierce it with a fork.

Carb Cycling with Sweet Potatoes

Each of the three carb cycles was designed specifically to burn fat like crazy…as long as you eat healthy, whole foods from as close to nature as possible, most of the time. You will not only see results, more importantly, you will sustain them.

The Sweet Potato Diet's meal plan has been built using natural, whole foods to help you:

- Keep your metabolism soaring, ensuring you not only lose weight faster, but maintain that weight loss for the long haul.
- Maintain better energy levels, so you stay energized and ready to give more during every workout.
- Ensure you feel good and emotionally well, reducing food cravings and temptation.

The Sweet Potato Diet's nutrition plan looks like this:

- Lean meats, fish, and poultry
- Veggies
- Fruit
- Roots and tubers
- Nuts and seeds

No sugar or alcohol. I know it's a bummer. Get through at least 30 days and then treat yourself to a glass of wine.

Included at the end of this book is an easy-to-use approved foods list and grocery guide and an excellent sweet potato recipe guide loaded with step-by-step recipes and directions on how to enjoy them on your carb cycle.

- All the allowed foods are listed and included
- Any non-approved foods have been excluded

Don't worry, the list is huge, so you won't find it difficult to find foods you love. And now it's super easy for you to pick delicious, healthy, fat-burning food and meals. All the recipes provide high-quality nutrition.

It's literally all done for you. So be sure to take your grocery guides and meal planner with you when you hit the aisles.

Approved Foods and Grocery Guide

VEGETABLES, ROOTS AND TUBERS

- ☐ ARTICHOKES
- ☐ ASPARAGUS
- ☐ BEETS
- ☐ BOK CHOY
- ☐ BROCCOLI
- ☐ BROWN POTATOES
- ☐ BRUSSEL SPROUTS
- ☐ BUTTERNUT SQUASH
- ☐ CAULIFLOWER
- ☐ CABBAGE
- ☐ CARROTS
- ☐ CELERY
- ☐ CUCUMBERS
- ☐ EGGPLANT
- ☐ GREEN BEANS
- ☐ GREEN BELL PEPPERS
- ☐ KALE
- ☐ MUSHROOMS
- ☐ ONIONS
- ☐ PARSNIPS
- ☐ RED BELL PEPPERS
- ☐ RED POTATOES
- ☐ ROMAINE LETTUCE
- ☐ SNAP PEAS
- ☐ SPINACH
- ☐ SWEET POTATOES
- ☐ SWISS CHARD
- ☐ YELLOW BELL PEPPERS

FRUITS

- ☐ APPLES
- ☐ APRICOTS
- ☐ AVOCADOS
- ☐ BANANAS [SPARINGLY]
- ☐ BLACKBERRIES
- ☐ BLUEBERRIES
- ☐ CANTALOUPES
- ☐ CHERRIES
- ☐ DATES [SPARINGLY]
- ☐ FIGS
- ☐ GUAVAS
- ☐ GRAPEFRUITS
- ☐ GRAPES
- ☐ HONEYDEW MELONS
- ☐ KIWIS
- ☐ LEMONS
- ☐ LIMES
- ☐ LYCHEE
- ☐ MANGOS
- ☐ ORANGES
- ☐ PAPAYAS
- ☐ PEACHES
- ☐ PEARS
- ☐ PINEAPPLES
- ☐ PLUMS
- ☐ POMEGRANATES
- ☐ RASPBERRIES
- ☐ STRAWBERRIES
- ☐ ROMA TOMATOES
- ☐ CHERRY TOMATOES
- ☐ WATERMELONS

FATS

- ☐ AVOCADO OIL
- ☐ COCONUT OIL
- ☐ GRASS-FED BUTTER
- ☐ GHEE
- ☐ BACON FAT/LARD
- ☐ DUCK FAT
- ☐ OLIVE OIL
- ☐ MACADAMIA OIL
- ☐ TALLOW
- ☐ WALNUT OIL

[Continued on next page]

BEVERAGES

- ☐ ALMOND MILK
- ☐ COCONUT MILK
- ☐ COCONUT WATER
- ☐ RAW MILK
- ☐ ORGANIC WHOLE MILK
- ☐ FLAX MILK
- ☐ TEA
- ☐ KOMBUCHA
- ☐ WATER (MINERAL, SPARKLING, FILTERED)

NUTS & SEEDS

- ☐ ALMONDS
- ☐ BRAZIL NUTS
- ☐ CASHEWS
- ☐ HAZELNUTS
- ☐ MACADAMIA NUTS
- ☐ PECANS
- ☐ PINE NUTS
- ☐ PISTACHIOS
- ☐ PUMPKIN SEEDS
- ☐ QUINOA
- ☐ SESAME SEEDS
- ☐ SUNFLOWER SEEDS
- ☐ WALNUTS

MEAT & POULTRY

- ☐ BACON
- ☐ BEEF (80% LEAN)
- ☐ BEEF (90% LEAN)
- ☐ STEAK
- ☐ BISON
- ☐ CHICKEN
- ☐ TURKEY
- ☐ DUCK
- ☐ LAMB
- ☐ PORK
- ☐ VEAL
- ☐ VENISON

SEAFOOD

- ☐ CATFISH
- ☐ CLAMS
- ☐ CRAB
- ☐ HALIBUT
- ☐ LOBSTER
- ☐ MAHI MAHI
- ☐ MUSSELS
- ☐ OYSTERS
- ☐ SALMON
- ☐ SARDINES
- ☐ SCALLOPS
- ☐ SHRIMP
- ☐ TUNA
- ☐ TROUT
- ☐ SEA BASS

KITCHEN STAPLES

- ☐ ALMOND FLOUR
- ☐ COCONUT FLOUR
- ☐ NUT BUTTERS (EXLUDING PEANUT)
- ☐ SALSA
- ☐ BROTHS (HOMEMADE FROM CHICKEN, BEEF, OR VEGGIES)
- ☐ KETCHUP
- ☐ FAT-FREE MAYO
- ☐ MUSTARD
- ☐ PICKLES
- ☐ LIME JUICE
- ☐ LEMON JUICE

SUPPLEMENTS

- ☐ PROBIOTICS (UNLESS YOU EAT FERMENTED VEGETABLES OR DRINK KOMBUCHA)
- ☐ WHEY PROTEIN (GRASS-FED IF POSSIBLE, OTHERWISE AN ISOLATE)
- ☐ COD LIVER OR KRILL OIL
- ☐ MCT OIL
- ☐ VITAMIN D

EGGS

- ☐ CHICKEN EGGS
- ☐ DUCK EGGS
- ☐ GOOSE EGGS
- ☐ QUAIL EGGS
- ☐ TURKEY EGGS

GRAINS

- ☐ WHITE RICE
- ☐ EZEKIEL BREAD
- ☐ OATS (ORGANIC STEEL CUT)
- ☐ COUSCOUS

DAIRY

- ☐ GREEK YOGURT
- ☐ FETA CHEESE
- ☐ MOZZARELLA CHEESE
- ☐ GOAT CHEESE

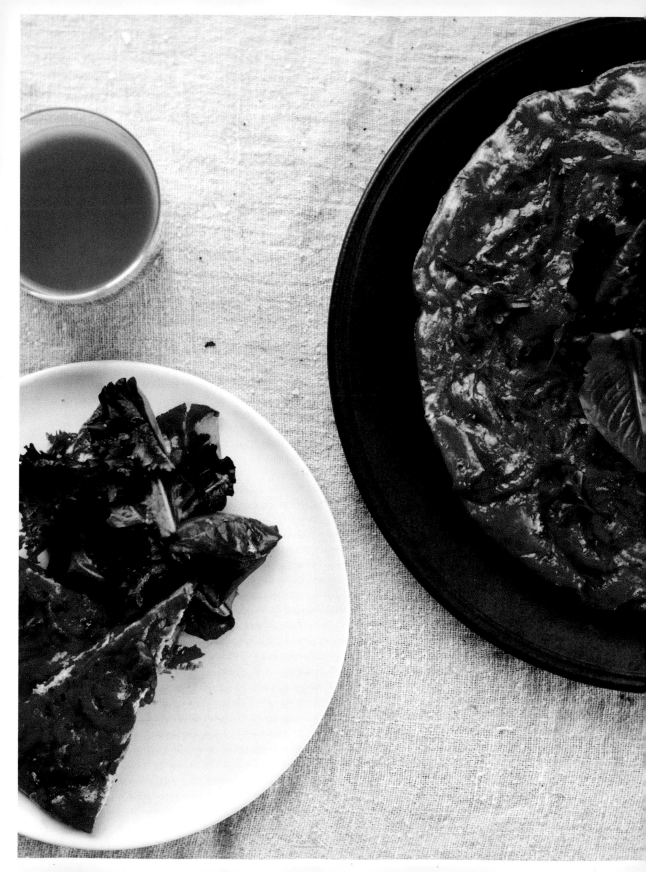

CHAPTER 11:

Breakfast: 8 Recipes

B reakfast is the perfect time for the sweet potato. I mean, any time is sweet potato time, haha, and just wait until you give the hash a go! Damn, that's all I've got to say. Nothing like waking up to the sweet smell of sweet potato hash. Not to mention, starting your day with these both satisfying and healthy meals will lead to you staying fuller longer and energized throughout the day.

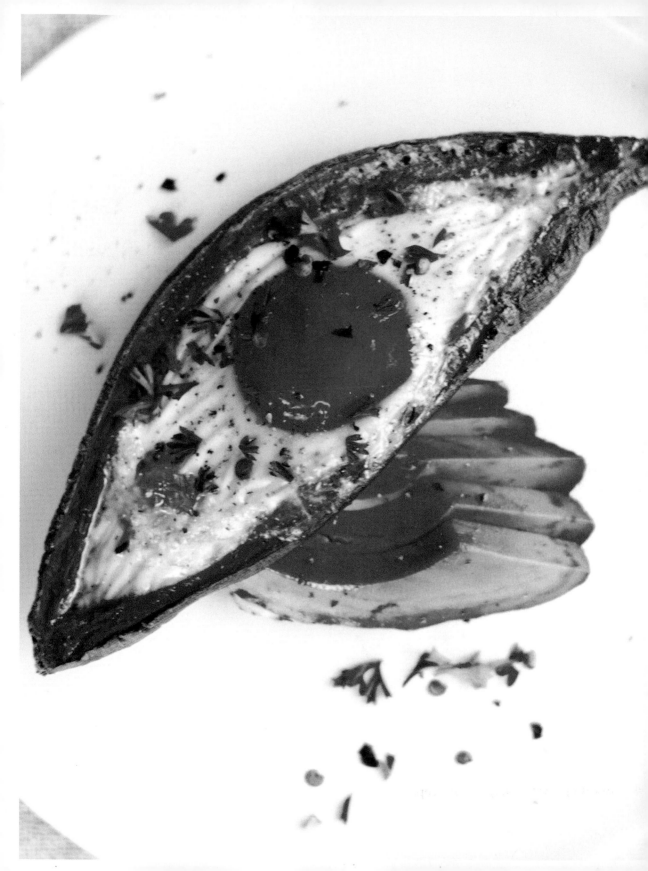

Baked Egg and Sweet Potato

Prep time: 5 minutes | Cook time: 20 minutes | Serves 2

Eggs are one of the best breakfast foods to get high-quality fats and protein into your system. This Baked Egg and Sweet Potato recipe revs up your metabolism and sets you up for success for the rest of the day.

1 sweet potato, cooked

2 eggs

1 tbsp butter

1. Cook sweet potato in the microwave (around 5 minutes) until soft.
2. Once cooled, cut in half. Scoop out the middle, leaving a good edge of sweet potato.
3. Add ½ tbsp butter to each half.
4. Add 1 egg to each half.
5. Heat oven to 350° F. Bake halves 15 minutes.

Calories 182 | Carbs 14g | Fat 11g | Protein 7g

HOW TO USE IT IN YOUR SWEET POTATO CYCLE

This meal serves as 1 serving of carbs and 1–2 servings of fat. Feel free to count the protein as ½ of your intake.

NOTE: *If you grab and use a sweet potato the size of your fist, you can be sure it's one serving of carbs.*

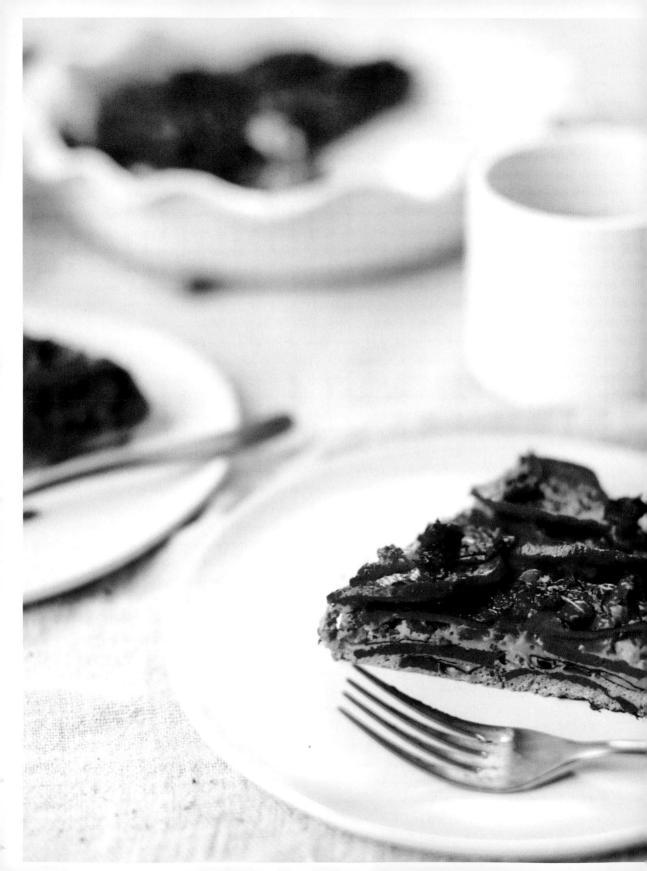

Breakfast Casserole

Prep time: 20 minutes | Cook time: 30 minutes | Serves 6

This amazing one dish wonder keeps breakfast not only simple to make, but simple to clean up. Use the sausage of your liking to bring either a sweet or spicy taste to this dish.

1 sweet potato, peeled and sliced

½ lb sausage, cooked

1 small onion, diced

1 cup spinach, chopped

6 eggs, beaten

1. Preheat oven to 375° F.
2. Layer all ingredients, except eggs, in a 9x9 baking dish.
3. Pour eggs over the top.
4. Bake 25–30 minutes or until eggs are cooked through.

Calories 340 | Carbs 26g | Fat 17g | Protein 28g

HOW TO USE IT IN YOUR SWEET POTATO CYCLE

This meal serves as 1 serving of carbs, 2 servings of fat, and 2 servings of protein.

NOTE: If you grab and use a sweet potato the size of your fist, you can be sure it's one serving of carbs.

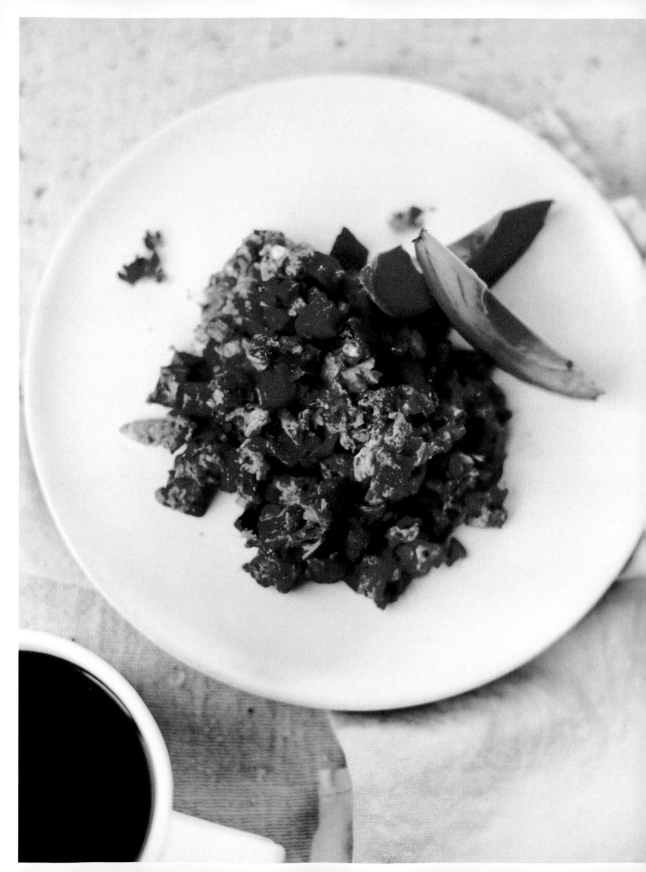

Sweet Potato Breakfast Hash

Prep time: 10 minutes | Cook time: 25 minutes | Serves 2

Potato hash is a breakfast classic loved by so many people. But, this time we are changing it up with the sweet taste of the sweet potato. Turkey sausage is a great source of protein to make this dish filling.

1 medium sweet potato, cubed

¼ lb turkey sausage

3 eggs, beaten

1. Cook sausage in a skillet until done, then set aside.
2. Add sweet potato and onion to skillet and cook until sweet potato is tender.
3. Add sausage and egg. Cook until egg is no longer runny.

Calories 285 | Carbs 21g | Fat 12g | Protein 22g

HOW TO USE IT IN YOUR SWEET POTATO CYCLE

This meal serves as 1 serving of carbs and 1 serving of fat, and about ¾ serving of protein.

NOTE: *If you grab and use a sweet potato the size of your fist, you can be sure it's one serving of carbs.*

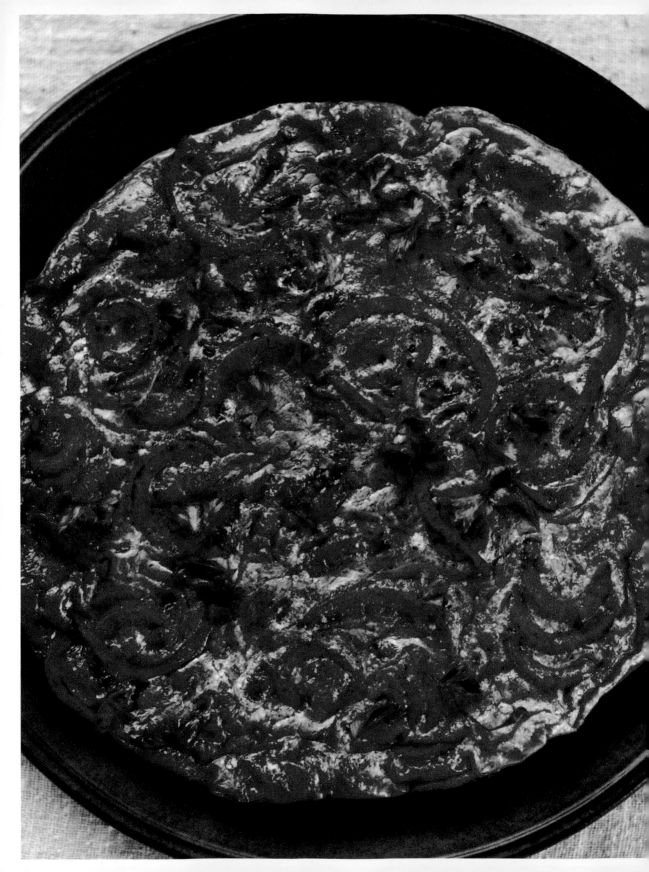

Sweet Potato Frittata

Prep time: 10 minutes | Cook time: 10 minutes | Serves 2

The frittata is an egg-based dish with the likeness of an open-faced omelet. Spiralized sweet potatoes bring a new twist to this dish, as they brighten the taste and add a slightly sweet note to the savory eggs.

1 sweet potato, peeled and spiraled

6 eggs, beaten

pinch of salt

pepper to taste

1. Spray an oven-safe skillet with coconut oil.
2. Over medium-high heat, add sweet potato. Let cook for a few minutes until color becomes brighter.
3. Reduce heat to medium-low and add eggs. Let this cook for several minutes.
4. Carefully lift the corner of the eggs to check for a golden brown color.
5. Once the bottom of the eggs is golden brown, turn off heat and place the pan under a broiler until top of eggs becomes golden brown.

Calories 328 | Carbs 15g | Fat 20g | Protein 21g

HOW TO USE IT IN YOUR SWEET POTATO CYCLE

This meal serves as 1 serving of carbs and 2 servings of fat, and about ¾ serving of protein.

NOTE: If you grab and use a sweet potato the size of your fist, you can be sure it's one serving of carbs.

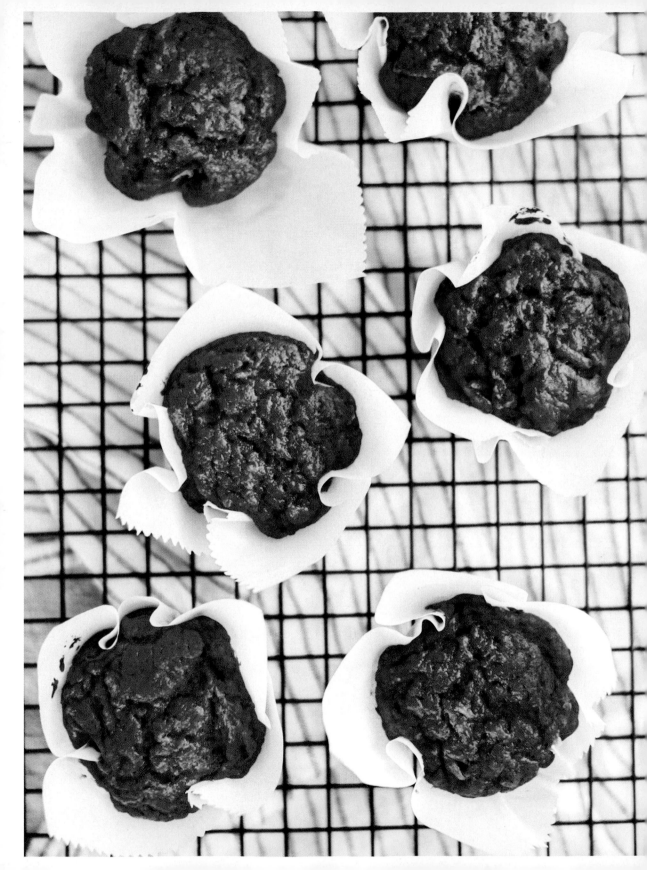

Sweet Potato Muffins

Prep time: 15 minutes | Cook time: 15 minutes | Makes 12 muffins

Muffins are an easy grab-and-go breakfast for anyone pressed for time in the morning. They also make great snacks to take along with you anywhere. These sweet potato muffins are a perfect breakfast treat.

1 cup sweet potato, mashed

1 apple, shredded

½ cup maple syrup

2 eggs

2 tbsp butter, melted

1 tsp vanilla

1 cup flour

1 ½ tsp baking soda

½ tsp salt

1 tsp cinnamon

¼ tsp nutmeg

1. Preheat oven to 375° F.
2. Mix wet ingredients in one bowl.
3. Mix dry ingredients in another bowl.
4. Fold dry ingredients into wet ingredients.
5. Spoon batter into lined muffin tin and fill ⅔ full.
6. Bake 15 minutes.

Calories 114 | Carbs 20g | Fat 3g | Protein 2g

HOW TO USE IT IN YOUR SWEET POTATO CYCLE

This meal serves as 1 serving of carbs.

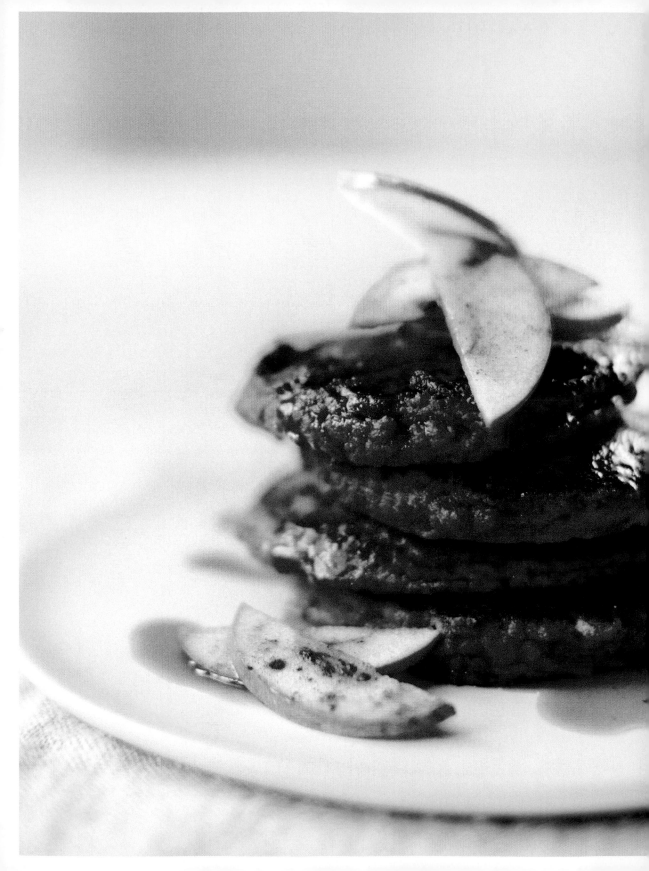

Sweet Potato Protein Pancakes

Prep time: 10 minutes | Cook time: 20 minutes | Serves 6

Pancakes are an all-time breakfast favorite. These pancakes are quick and simple and are also a favorite with the kids. This recipe uses coconut to add an extra dessert-like flavor to this unique pancake.

½ cup mashed sweet potato

1 cup protein powder

1 cup coconut or almond milk

¼ cup coconut flour

1 egg

½ cup applesauce

1 tsp. cinnamon

1 tsp. baking soda

1 tsp. baking powder

1 tsp. arrowroot starch

1. Combine all ingredients.
2. Cook in a skillet until sides begin to look dry, flip, then continue to cook until done.

Calories 158 | Carbs 15g | Fat 4g | Protein 14g

HOW TO USE IT IN YOUR SWEET POTATO CYCLE

This meal serves as 1–1½ servings of carbs.

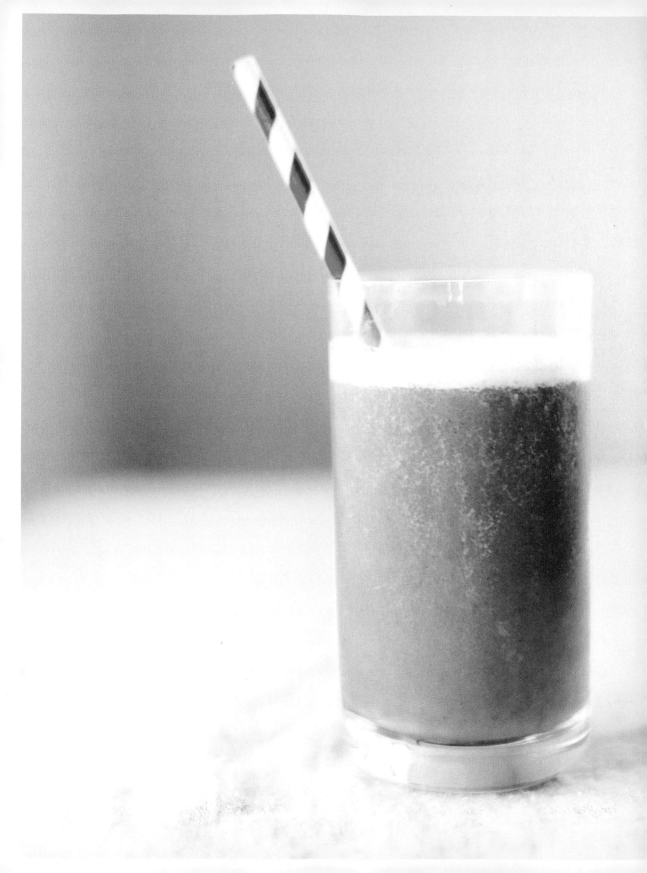

Sweet Potato Smoothie

Prep time: 5 minutes | Serves 1

Smoothies are a great way to start your morning. These blend up into a delicious and creamy—not to mention very portable—breakfast. A bit of cinnamon and vanilla make this smoothie a one-of-a-kind sweet potato experience.

½ cup freshly squeezed orange juice

½ cup coconut milk

¼ cup sweet potato, cooked

1 tsp vanilla

¼ tsp cinnamon

1 scoop Morellifit Nutrition Vanilla Protein

1 handful of ice

Just one step: Place all ingredients in a blender and puree.

Calories 230 | Carbs 24g | Fat 4g | Protein 22g

HOW TO USE IT IN YOUR SWEET POTATO CYCLE

This meal serves as 1½ servings of carbs and about ½ serving of protein.

*NOTE: *If you grab and use a sweet potato the size of your fist, you can be sure it's one serving of carbs.*

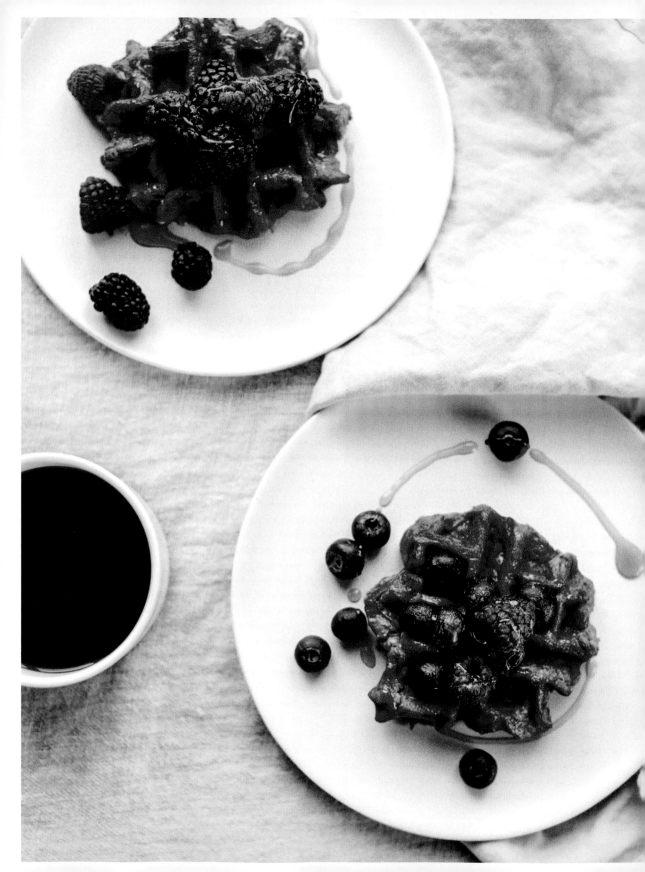

Sweet Potato Waffles

Prep time: 15 minutes | Cook time: 20 minutes | Serves 3

Everyone loves waffles! And now you can enjoy them guilt-free. In fact, these are just as filling, yet don't sit like a brick at the bottom off your belly as most waffles do. You can enjoy them with or without syrup, it all depends on what day of your cycle you happen to be on.

  1 small sweet potato, peeled and spiraled

  1 cup mashed sweet potato

  2 eggs, beaten

  3 tbsp coconut milk

  1 tsp cinnamon

1. Mix all ingredients together.
2. Spray the waffle iron with coconut spray and preheat.
3. Drop ½ cup onto the waffle maker.
4. Cook until outside is crispy.

Calories 130 | Carbs 19g | Fat 4g | Protein 19g

HOW TO USE IT IN YOUR SWEET POTATO CYCLE

This meal serves as 1–1½ servings of carbs.

NOTE: If you grab and use a sweet potato the size of your fist, you can be sure it's one serving of carbs.

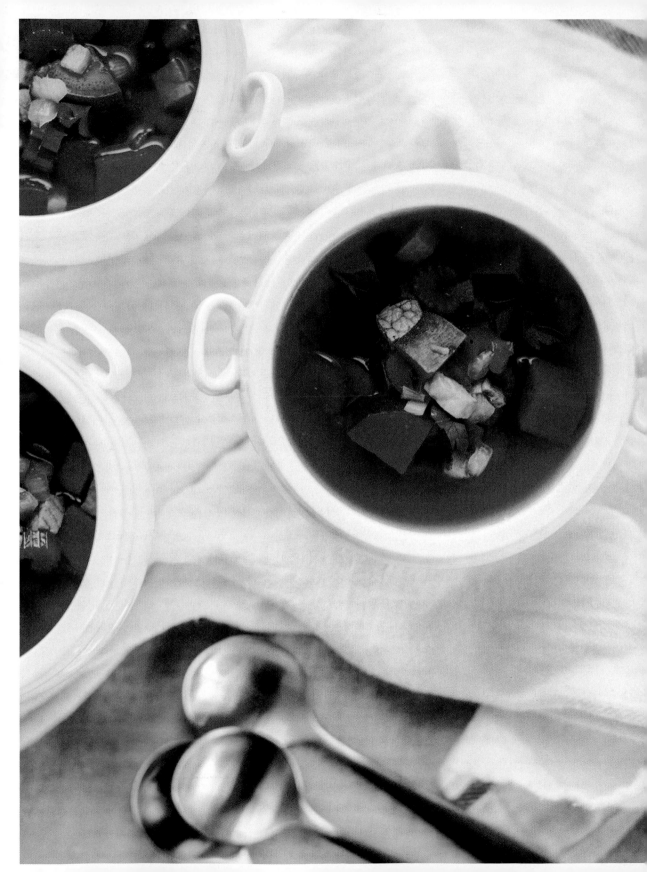

CHAPTER 12:

Soups: 5 Recipes

love soup, especially homemade. A good bowl of soup can really hit the spot, and sweet potatoes only make it better. Whether added to your soup or blended for a creamy base, the texture of the sweet potato easily makes it one of the best for soup.

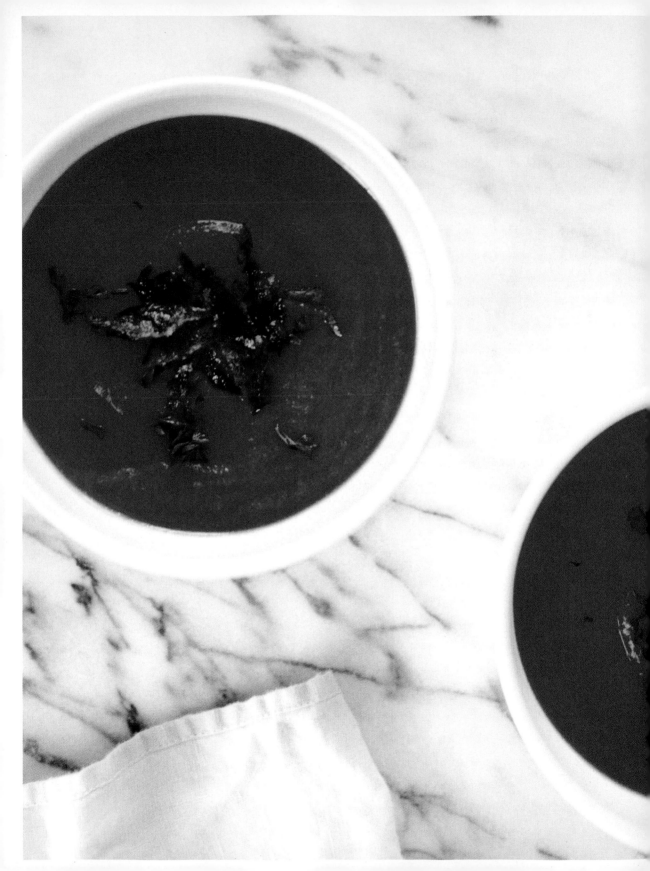

Cauliflower and Bacon Soup

Prep time: 20 minutes | Cook time: 4 hours | Serves 8

The bacon in this recipe adds an extra layer of smoky flavor to the sweet potato and cauliflower that is simply irresistible. This is a simple recipe that you will want to make again and again. Plus, the crockpot is the ultimate cooking time saver.

2 small sweet potatoes, peeled and chopped

6 cups water

2 tbsp chicken bouillon

1 can coconut milk

3 cloves garlic

1 tsp salt

1. Place all ingredients in a crockpot and cook on high for 4 hours.
2. Using an immersion blender, blend the soup until smooth.

Calories 260 | Carbs 16g | Fat 20g | Protein 7g

HOW TO USE IT IN YOUR SWEET POTATO CYCLE

This meal serves as 1 serving of carbs and 2 servings of fat.

NOTE: If you grab and use a sweet potato the size of your fist, you can be sure it's one serving of carbs.

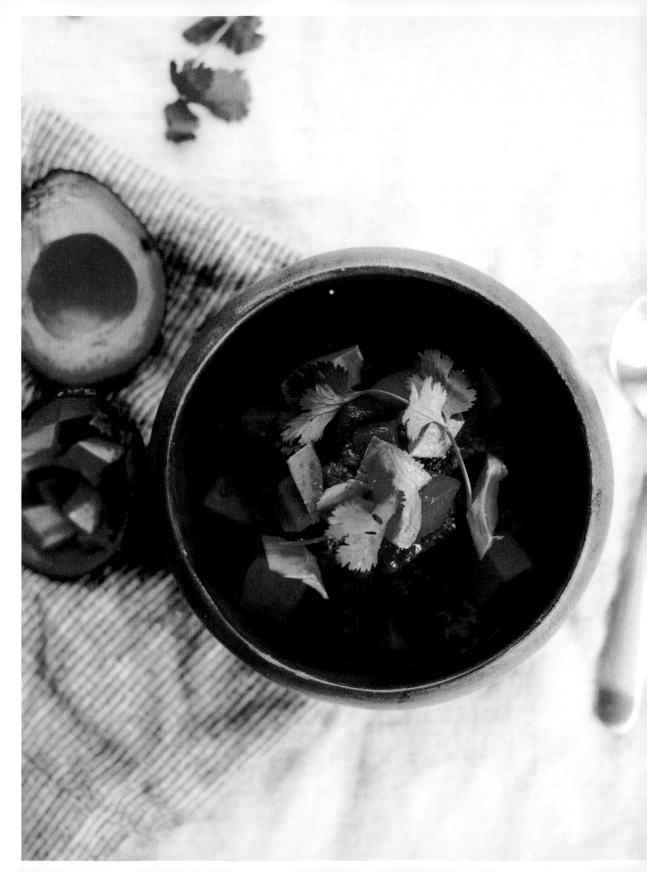

Sweet Potato Chili

Prep time: 15 minutes | Cook time: 30 minutes | Serves 6

Everybody loves a good bowl of chili, and with sweet potatoes, this classic favorite just got even better. Not only is it good for you, giving you all the benefits of the sweet potato, but it is oh so delicious, too!

1 lb ground beef

1 medium onion, chopped

1 bell or poblano pepper, seeded
   and chopped

1 jalapeno, seeded and chopped

1 tbsp chili powder

1 tsp oregano

1 tsp salt

½ tsp cumin

2 cups sweet potatoes, diced

1 can tomato sauce

1 can diced tomato

½ cup water

1. In a heavy-bottomed pot, add ground beef, onion, peppers, jalapeno, chili powder, oregano, salt, and cumin.
2. Cook everything together until beef is cooked through, then add the remaining ingredients.
3. Simmer until potatoes are soft.

Calories 260 | Carbs 31g | Fat 8g | Protein 20g

HOW TO USE IT IN YOUR SWEET POTATO CYCLE

This meal serves as 2 servings of carbs, 1 serving of fat, and 1 serving of protein.

NOTE: *If you grab and use a sweet potato the size of your fist, you can be sure it's one serving of carbs.*

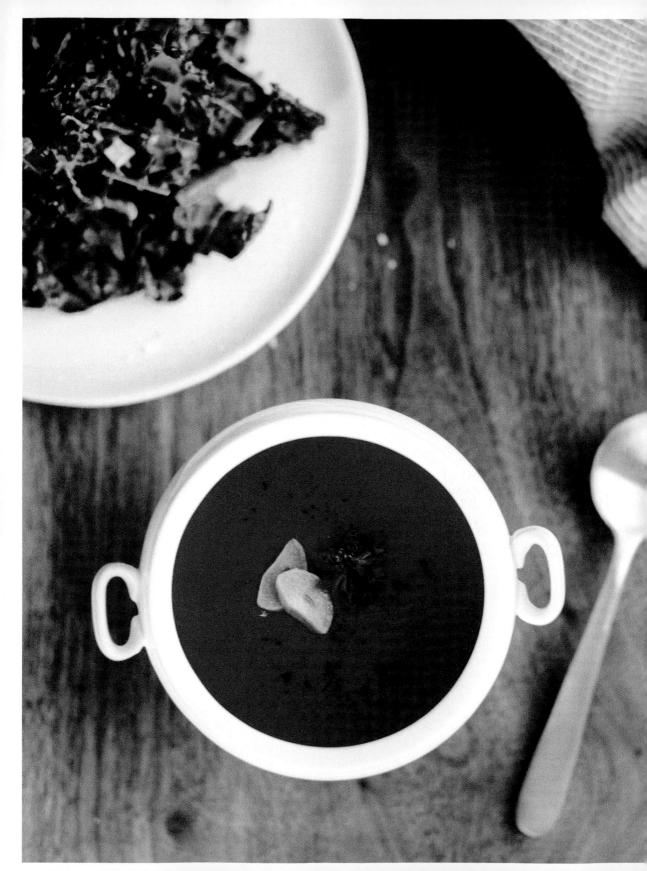

Curried Sweet Potato Soup

Prep time: 5 minutes | Cook time: 20 minutes | Serves 4

This curried sweet potato soup is the perfect comfort on a cold day and makes amazing leftovers so you can keep on enjoying it as a quick grab-and-go meal.

1 large sweet potato, peeled and cubed

1 medium onion, quartered

4 cloves garlic, whole

1 can coconut milk

2 cups chicken broth

2 tbsp curry powder

1. Preheat oven to 425° F.
2. On a baking sheet lined with parchment paper, place sweet potato, onion, and garlic cloves, then spray with coconut oil.
3. Bake in oven until sweet potatoes are tender.
4. Place veggies in a saucepan with coconut milk, broth, and curry powder.
5. Let it simmer until hot.
6. VERY CAREFULLY use an immersion blender to puree the soup. If you don't have an immersion blender, very carefully pour soup into a blender and pulse until smooth.

Calories 200 | Carbs 17g | Fat 12g | Protein 5g

HOW TO USE IT IN YOUR SWEET POTATO CYCLE

This meal serves as 1 serving of carbs and 1 serving of fat. You can count the protein if you'd like, but it's minimal, so make sure to get some more to satisfy the requirements.

NOTE: If you grab and use a sweet potato the size of your fist, you can be sure it's one serving of carbs.

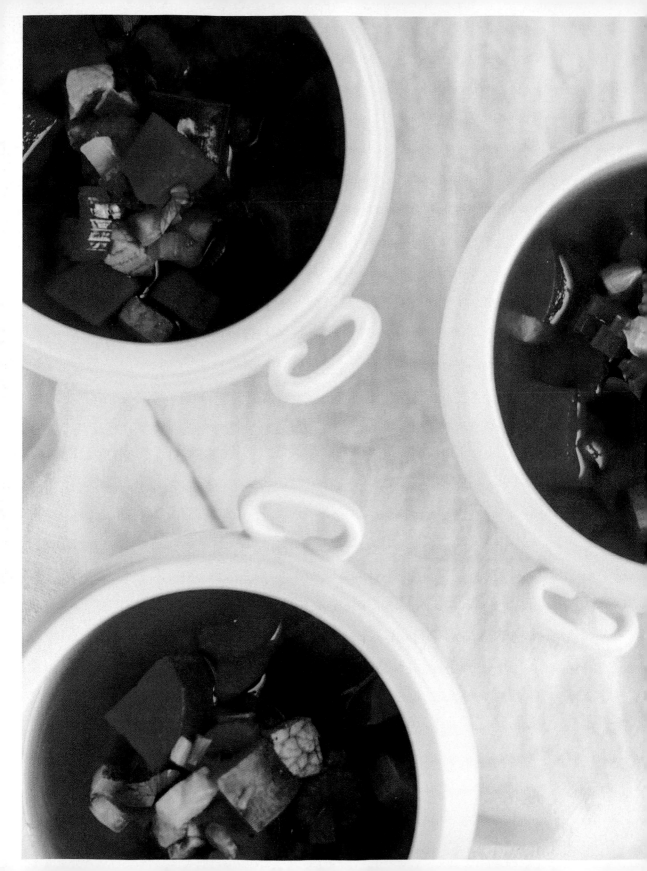

Ham and Sweet Potato Stew

Prep time: 10 minutes | Cook time: 60 minutes | Serves 6

There are so many different ways to make a stew, each recipe containing its own unique blend of meats and veggies, that it has become an art. This masterpiece brings together ham and sweet potato for an amazing blend of flavors that is sure to please everyone.

1 lb smoked ham, cubed

½ cup onion, diced

½ cup celery, diced

1 medium sweet potato, cut into ½ inch cubes

6 cups water

1 tsp salt

1 tsp black pepper

1 tsp dried sage

1. Dice the vegetables and ham and add to a large sauce pan.
2. Cover with 6 cups water, add salt, pepper and sage.
3. Bring to a boil over medium heat, reduce to simmer and cook 1 hour.

Calories 125 | Carbs 12g | Fat 2g | Protein 14g

HOW TO USE IT IN YOUR SWEET POTATO CYCLE

This meal serves as 1 serving of carbs and about ⅓ serving of protein or a little bit less. Remember, you can always add more lean protein.

NOTE: If you grab and use a sweet potato the size of your fist, you can be sure it's one serving of carbs.

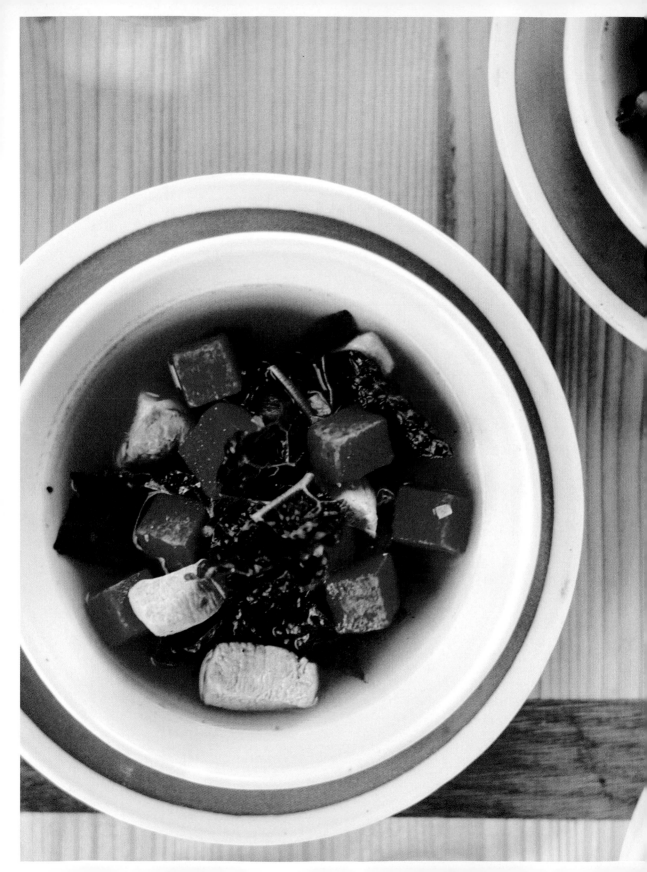

Chicken, Kale, and Sweet Potato Stew

Prep time: 20 minutes | Cook time: 90 minutes | Serves 4

Chicken soup is good for more than fighting off a cold. Our take on a simple dish will not only make you feel better when you're down but will help keep you healthy so you don't get sick In the first place. This soup-turned-stew makes a wonderful meal or side dish.

8 oz boneless, skinless chicken breast, cubed

1 small yellow onion, diced

3 cloves minced garlic

1 tbsp olive oil

3 cups cleaned and chopped kale

1 large sweet potato, cut in ½ inch cubes

6 cups chicken broth or water

salt and pepper to taste

1 sprig fresh rosemary

1. In a large, heavy pot, heat olive oil over medium heat.
2. Add chicken, onion, and garlic, and sauté 10 minutes until chicken is browned and onion is translucent. Add broth or water, stirring up any brown bits from the bottom.
3. Add remaining ingredients, reduce heat to low, and cover.
4. Let simmer for 45 minutes and check potato for tenderness. Simmer additional 15 minutes if needed.

Calories 171 | Carbs 14g | Fat 6g | Protein 15g

HOW TO USE IT IN YOUR SWEET POTATO CYCLE

This meal serves as 1 serving of carbs (little less) and ½ a serving of fat. Add more protein to each serving to satisfy your requirements for the the day of your cycle.

*NOTE: *If you grab and use a sweet potato the size of your fist, you can be sure it's one serving of carbs.*

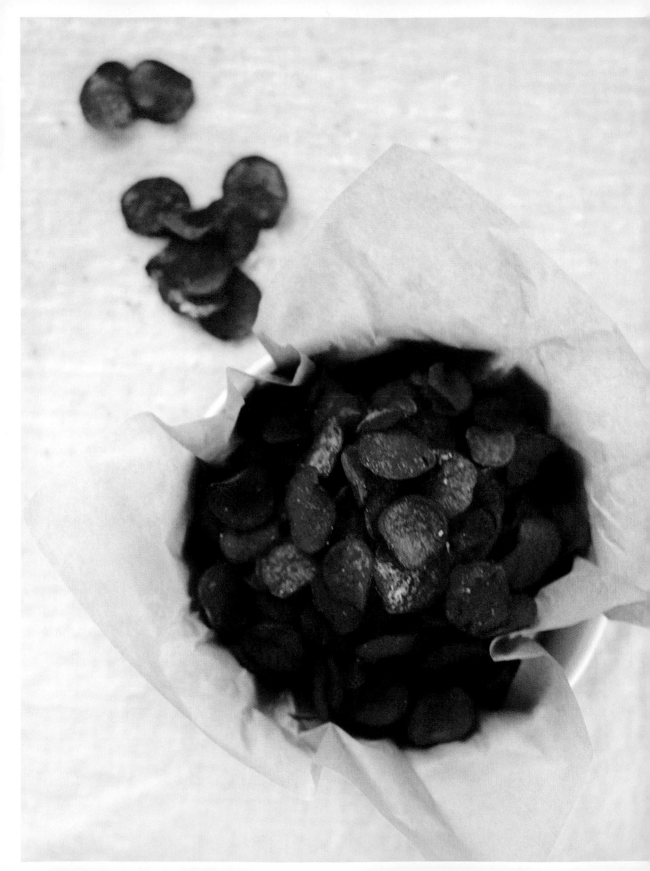

CHAPTER 13:

Sides: 7 Recipes

S weet potatoes go great with everything (at least I think so, haha!), which means they are great for sides. And with so many ways to prepare the sweet potato, these sides never get boring (just wait). Swap around your sides to meet the required cycle portions, or add them to some lean protein to keep things simple. I told you this wouldn't be a boring diet!

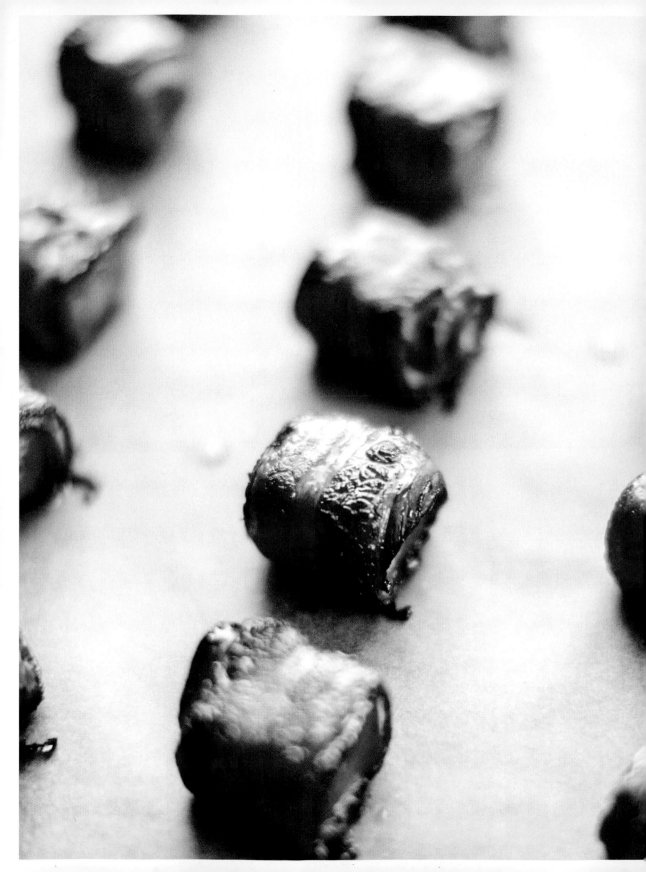

Bacon-Wrapped Sweet Potato

Prep time: 20 minutes | Cook time: 20 minutes | Serves 4

In this simple (yet mouthwatering) side dish, you have sweet potatoes that are wrapped in bacon...how can you possibly go wrong? The sweet of the honey and the hint of cayenne make this dish perfect.

2 small sweet potatoes, peeled and cubed

½ pound bacon

1 tbsp honey

1 tsp water

cayenne

1. Preheat oven to 400° F.
2. Wrap each sweet potato cube in bacon (toothpick optional to hold it all together).
3. Brush each with honey and water mixture. Sprinkle with cayenne.
4. Bake about 20 minutes or until bacon is crispy and sweet potatoes are soft.

Calories 163 | Carbs 18g | Fat 8g | Protein 9g

HOW TO USE IT IN YOUR SWEET POTATO CYCLE

This meal serves as 1½ servings of carbs, about 1 serving of fat, and a little less than ½ a serving of protein. Be careful not to add more bacon here, as the fat content will likely take you over the mark for healthy fats allowed. Instead, I would rather you add some leaner meat or egg whites.

*NOTE: *If you grab and use a sweet potato the size of your fist, you can be sure it's one serving of carbs.*

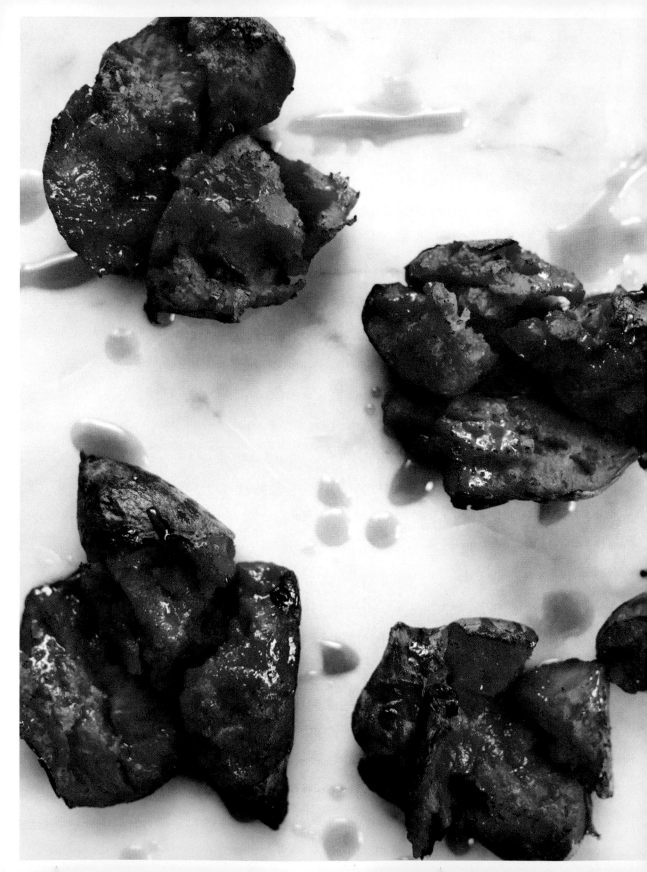

Crushed Sweet Potatoes

Prep time: 5 minutes | Cook time: 40 minutes | Serves 8

This side is deliciously sweet, simple, and fun to make. Using maple syrup is a great way to make the sweet potato even sweeter. And these will also be a pleasant surprise for those who are expecting traditional mashed potatoes.

4 small sweet potatoes

2 tbsp olive oil

salt

2 tbsp maple syrup

1. Place sweet potatoes on parchment paper-lined baking sheet and cut each in half.
2. Smash, not entirely, you want them to have a little thickness to them.
3. Drizzle each with oil, syrup, and salt.
4. Bake for 15 minutes.

Calories 201 | Carbs 17g | Fat 14g | Protein 1g

HOW TO USE IT IN YOUR SWEET POTATO CYCLE

This meal serves as 1 serving of carbs and 2 servings of fat.

*NOTE: If you grab and use a sweet potato the size of your fist, you can be sure it's one serving of carbs.

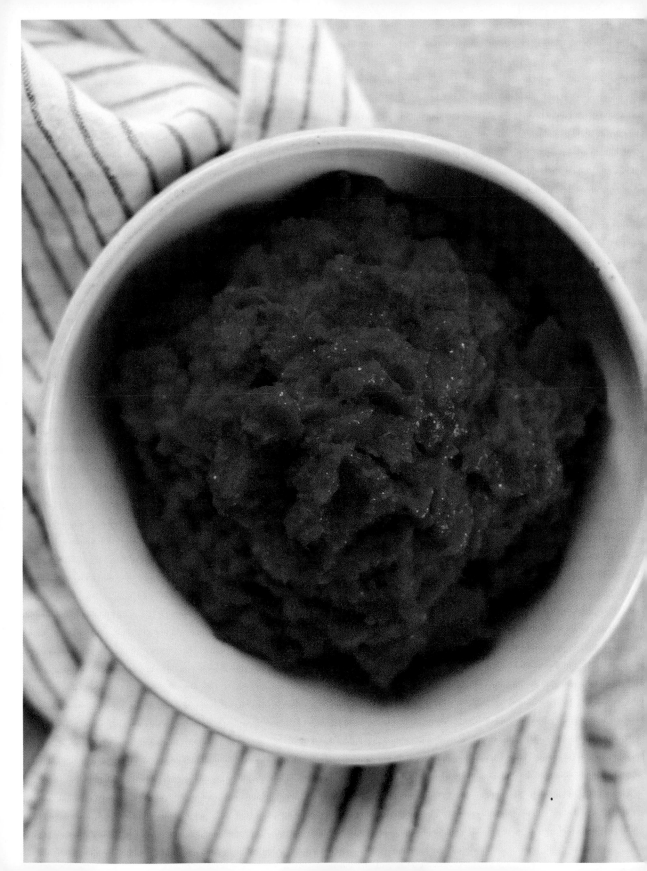

Mashed Sweet Potatoes

Prep time: 5 minutes | Cook time: 30 minutes | Serves 4

You can up your mashed potato game by using sweet potatoes and mixing them with Greek yogurt. This is a tasty way to make your potatoes even creamier. This is the perfect side choice for any dish.

2 tbsp butter

½ cup Greek yogurt (fat free)

1 tsp salt

pepper

1. Boil potatoes approximately 30 minutes, until tender when poked with a fork.
2. Drain and mash with all remaining ingredients.

Calories 160 | Carbs 21g | Fat 7g | Protein 11g

HOW TO USE IT IN YOUR SWEET POTATO CYCLE

This meal serves as 1½ servings of carbs, a serving of fat, and about ½ a serving of protein. If you're going to add more Greek yogurt here, just make sure it's fat free. Otherwise, you risk overdoing your fat intake for the meal.

NOTE: If you grab and use a sweet potato the size of your fist, you can be sure it's one serving of carbs.

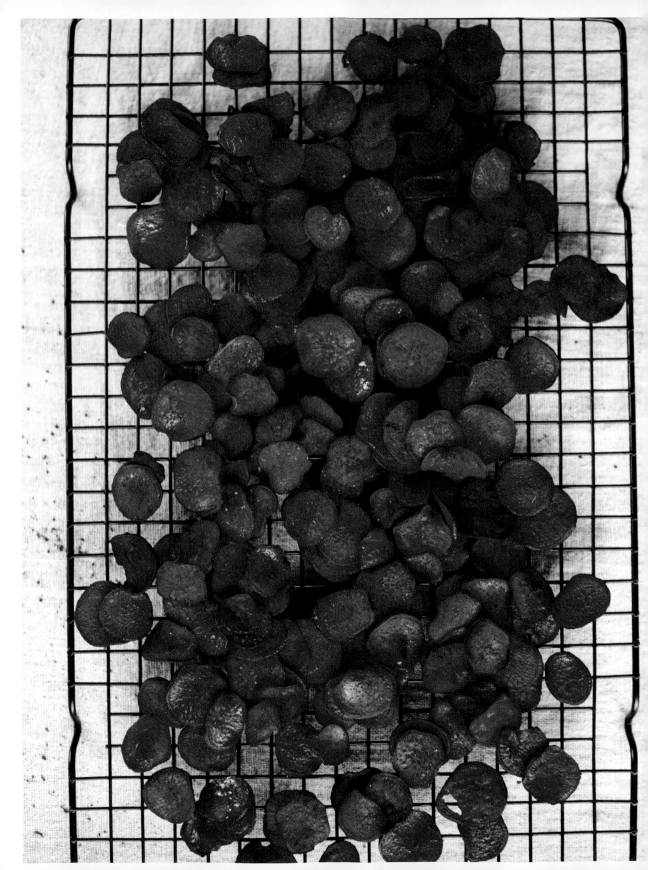

Sweet Potato Chips

Prep time: 5 minutes | Cook time: 20 minutes | Serves 2

Chips are a fun and tasty side for your lunch, but not always the healthiest choice. This recipe remedies that by using sweet potatoes and baking them instead of frying. Who doesn't love chips? These are the bomb!

1 medium sweet potato

1 tsp olive oil

salt

1. Preheat oven to 400° F.
2. Slice sweet potato thin. Try to get them all the same thickness.
3. Place sweet potatoes in a bowl and drizzle with olive oil.
4. Toss to coat the sweet potatoes evenly, then lay in a single layer on a baking sheet.
5. Cook for 20 minutes, turning after 10 minutes. Once cooked, sprinkle with salt.

Calories 80 | Carbs 13g | Fat 2g | Protein 1g

HOW TO USE IT IN YOUR SWEET POTATO CYCLE

This meal serves as 1 serving of carbs (a little less). Measure using your fist to get exactly what you need for your cycle. These are an easy way to add carbs to any meal.

NOTE: If you grab and use a sweet potato the size of your fist, you can be sure it's one serving of carbs.

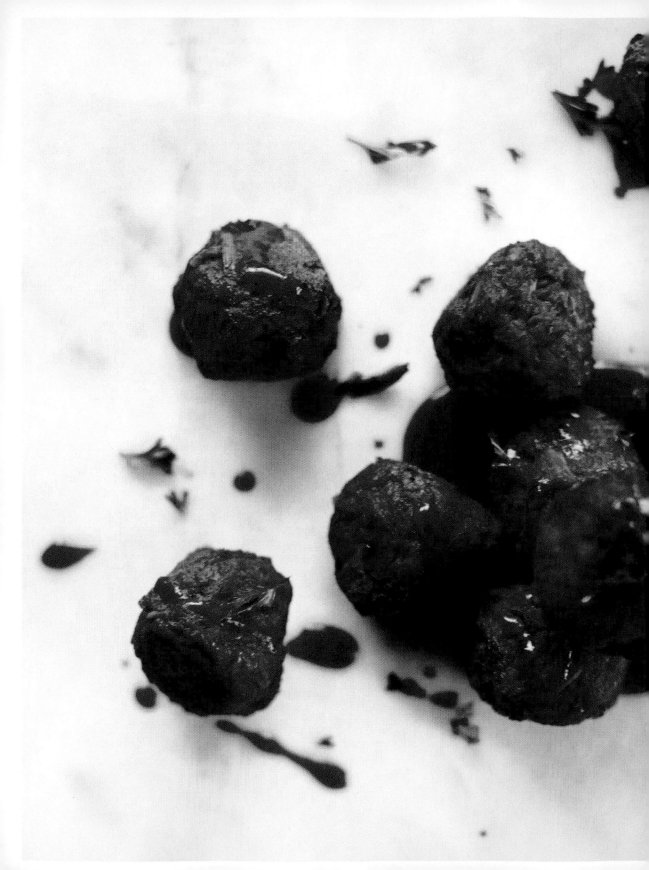

Sweet Potato Tots

Prep time: 15 minutes | Cook time: 15 minutes | Makes 25 tots (depending on tot size)

Tater tots are a fun side dish that go great with breakfast, lunch, and dinner. This recipe gives you an alternative to the traditional tots by making them healthier and tastier! Plus, these are a hit with kids and adults alike.

   1 small sweet potato, grated

   1 small sweet potato, mashed

   1 tbsp coconut flour

   ¼ tsp garlic salt

   ¼ tsp cayenne

   ¼ tsp paprika

   1 egg

   Frank's Red Hot hot sauce (if you like living on the edge, haha!)

1. Preheat oven to 350° F.
2. Combine ingredients except hot sauce and form into balls.
3. Line baking sheet with parchment paper and place tots on sheet.
4. Bake for 15 minutes, turning every 5 minutes.
5. Once out of the oven, coat with Frank's hot sauce while still warm.

Calories 90 | Carbs 15g | Fat 2g | Protein 3g

HOW TO USE IT IN YOUR SWEET POTATO CYCLE

This meal serves as about 1 serving of carbs, again, use your fist to make enough to satisfy your cycle's needs.

*NOTE: *If you grab and use a sweet potato the size of your fist, you can be sure it's one serving of carbs.*

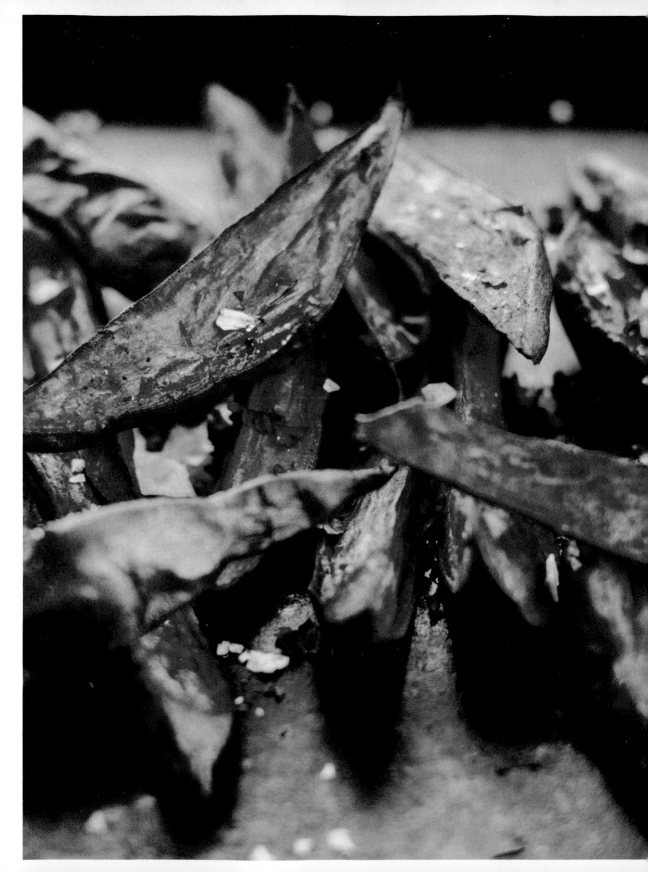

Sweet Potato Wedges

Prep time: 5 minutes | Cook time: 30–45 minutes | Serves 3

These sweet potato wedges are the perfect substitute for your classic potato wedges, and they pair nicely with the BBQ Chicken Burger in the next section. These wedges are a side that the whole family will love and are perfect for family gatherings.

4 small sweet potatoes

olive oil

paprika

garlic salt

salt & pepper

1. Preheat oven to 425° F.
2. Cut sweet potatoes into wedges and toss with olive oil and seasonings.
3. Line baking sheet with parchment paper.
4. Place wedges on lined baking sheet. Bake for 30-45 minutes or until wedges are soft.

Calories 140 | Carbs 28g | Fat 3g | Protein 2g

HOW TO USE IT IN YOUR SWEET POTATO CYCLE

This meal serves as 1½–2 servings of carbs.

__NOTE:__ If you grab and use a sweet potato the size of your fist, you can be sure it's one serving of carbs.

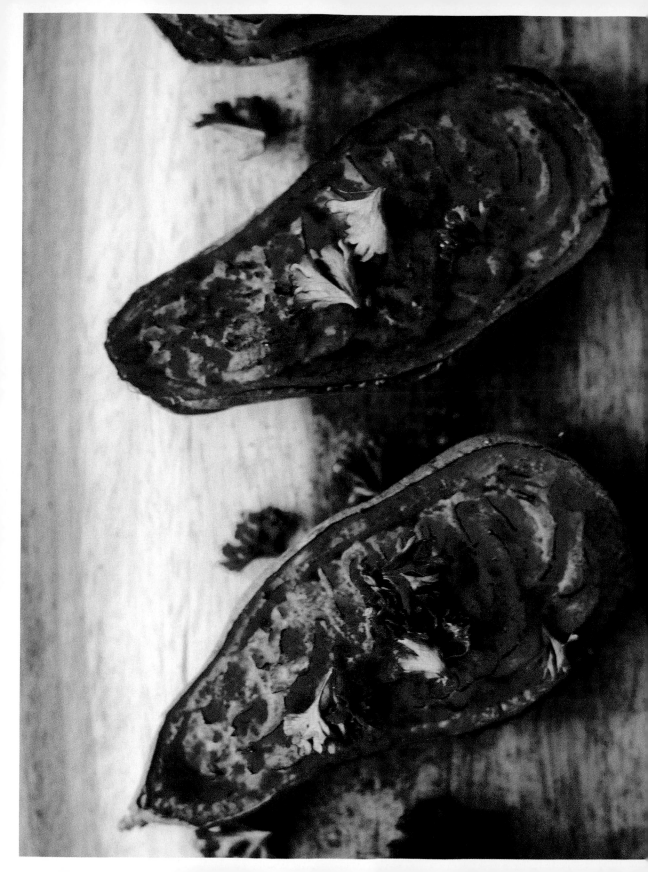

Twice-Baked Sweet Potatoes

Prep time: 20 minutes | Cook time: 45 minutes | Serves 4

Twice-baked sweet potatoes are a delicious side that you can pair with any dinner. The addition of Greek yogurt makes the sweet potato even creamier and even tastier. These potatoes are twice baked and twice as good as their classic counterparts.

2 medium sweet potatoes

½ cup Greek yogurt (fat free)

1 tbsp butter

½ tsp salt

½ tsp paprika

1. Scrub potatoes and bake at 350° F for about 30 minutes, or until tender.
2. Remove and let cool for 20 minutes, until easily handled.
3. Split each potato in half lengthwise and scoop out inside, leaving about ½ inch of potato attached to the skin.
4. Mix the scooped-out potato and mash with remaining ingredients until it's the consistency of mashed potato, then stuff reserved skins with the mixture.
5. Top with an additional sprinkle of paprika and bake 10–15 minutes at 350° F until lightly browned.

Calories 110 | Carbs 15g | Fat 4g | Protein 11g

HOW TO USE IT IN YOUR SWEET POTATO CYCLE

This meal serves as 1 serving of carbs, and about ½ a serving of protein. If you're going to add more Greek yogurt here make sure it's fat free, otherwise you risk overdoing your fat intake for the meal.

*NOTE: *If you grab and use a sweet potato the size of your fist, you can be sure it's one serving of carbs.*

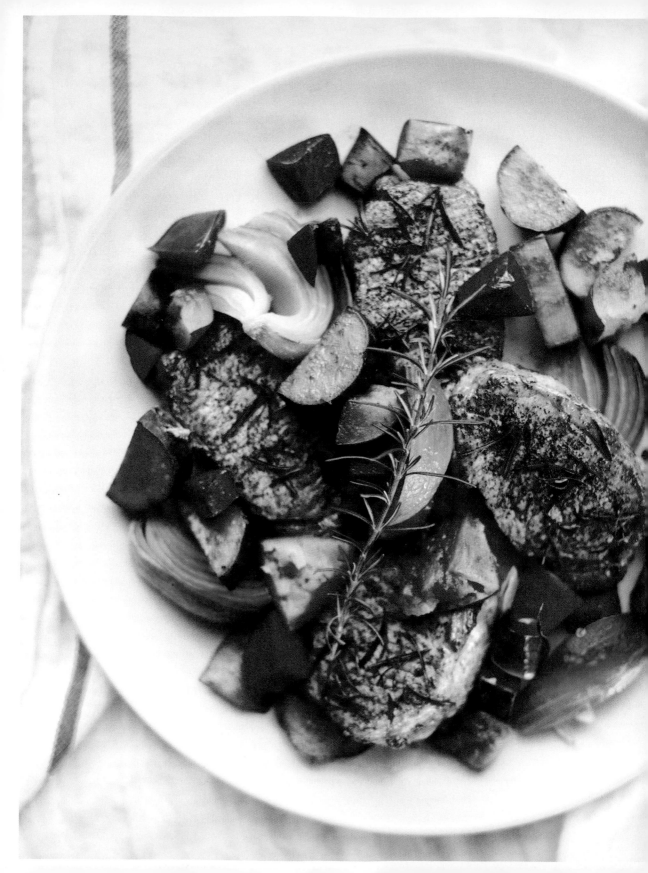

CHAPTER 14:

Dinner: 19 Recipes

D inner time and shortly after is when the cravings usually hit. Did you know your willpower diminishes the later it gets in the day? Seriously. Why do you think it's far more difficult to say no at night? It's important to eat a hearty and filling, and less calorie-dense meal if possible in the evening (depending on the cycle day of course). These dinner recipes are solid, and I am willing to bet you can get your entire family on board with these. Remember, make more and store for tomorrow. It's the easiest way (at least for me) to stay prepped.

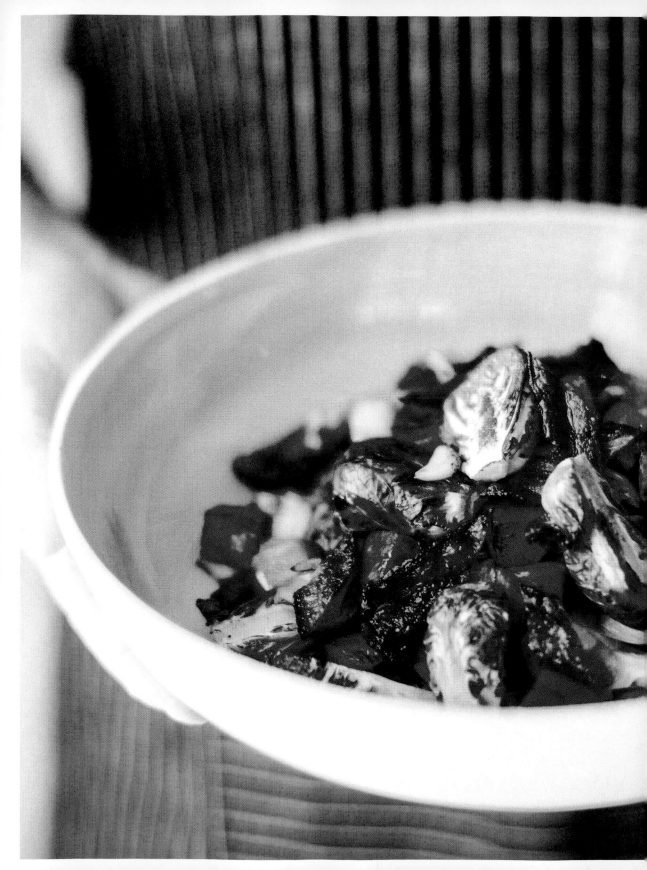

Bacon, Brussels Sprouts, and Sweet Potato

Prep time: 10 minutes | Cook time: 20 minutes | Serves 2

Brussels sprouts might be something you hid in your napkin as a kid, but not anymore. These succulent sprouts are tender and delicious and pair perfectly with the savory taste of bacon and sweet potato.

  1 large sweet potato

  1 lb Brussels sprouts

  1 small onion

  ½ lb bacon

  2 cloves garlic

  1 tsp coconut oil

  2 tsp balsamic vinegar

1. Preheat oven to 425° F.
2. Peel and cube potato into half-inch bites. Cut sprouts into fourths. Slice onion and chop bacon.
3. Toss all ingredients together to coat with oil and vinegar, then spread out on a baking sheet until evenly distributed.
4. Bake for 20 minutes until potatoes and Brussels sprouts are tender.

Calories 436 | Carbs 27g | Fat 25g | Protein 25g

HOW TO USE IT IN YOUR SWEET POTATO CYCLE

This meal serves as 1-2 servings of carbs, 2-3 servings of fat, and a serving of protein. This baby is very calorically dense!

NOTE: *If you grab and use a sweet potato the size of your fist, you can be sure it's one serving of carbs.*

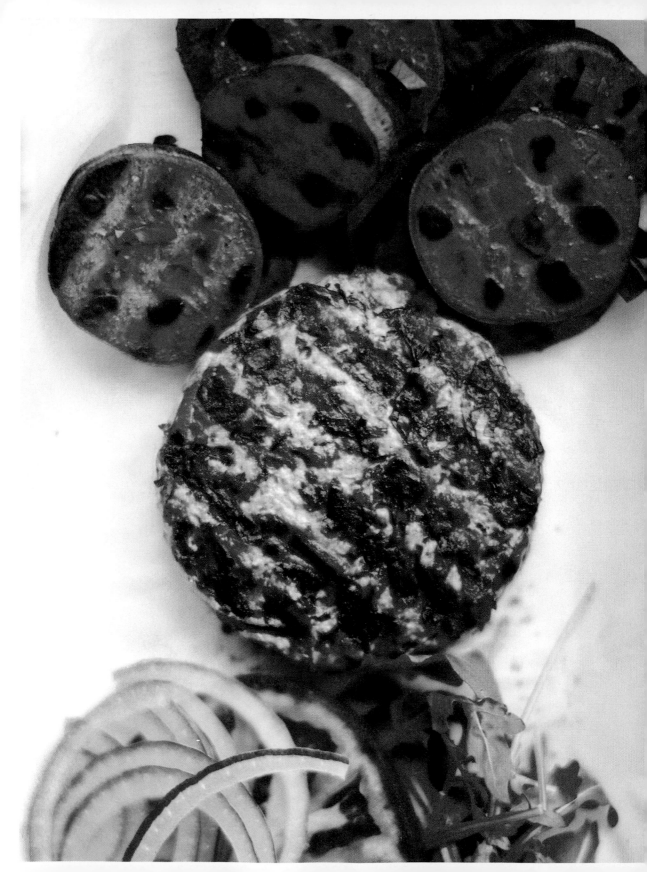

BBQ Chicken Burgers

Prep time: 10 minutes | Cook time: 20 minutes | Makes 4 burgers

These burgers are intentionally kept simple to allow for a variety of veggie toppings of your choice. Plus it makes these easy to make for lunch or dinner when you want to have a simple but delicious burger on the grill.

   1 lb ground chicken

   1 medium sweet potato, shredded

   1 cup spinach, chopped

   1 medium sweet potato, sliced thick

1. Mix the chicken, shredded sweet potato, and spinach, and form into patties.
2. Grill burgers; make sure the thermometer reads 175° F to ensure chicken is fully cooked.
3. Coat the sliced sweet potatoes with olive or coconut oil and place on grill until tender, flipping halfway through.
4. Top burger with sweet potato slices or serve on the side.

Calories 221 | Carbs 14g | Fat 9g | Protein 21g

HOW TO USE IT IN YOUR SWEET POTATO CYCLE

This meal serves as ¾-1 serving of carbs, a serving of fat, and about a serving of protein.

*NOTE: *If you grab and use a sweet potato the size of your fist, you can be sure it's one serving of carbs.*

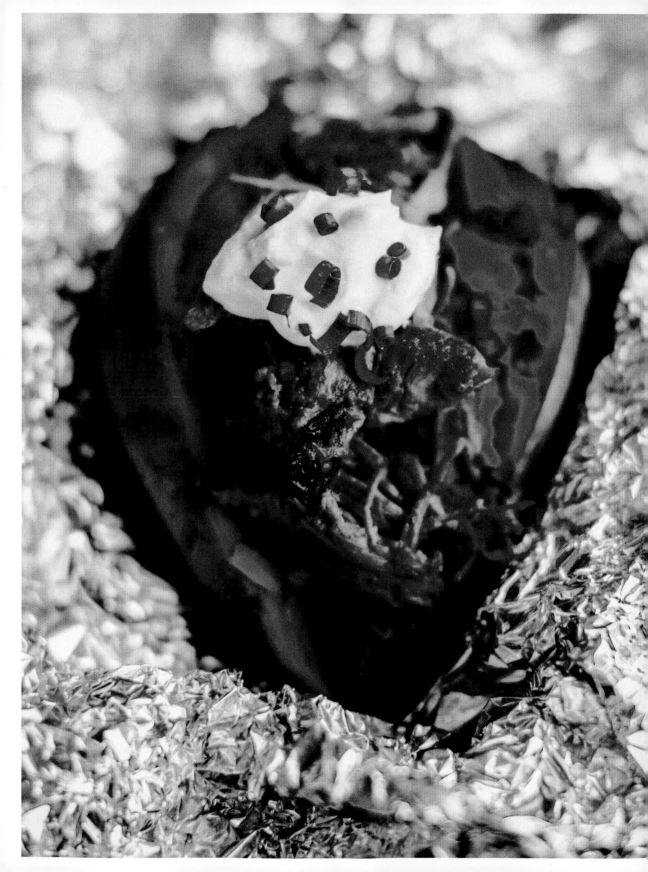

BBQ Pulled Pork Stuffed Potatoes

Prep time: 30 minutes | Cook time: 8 hours | Serves 6

This sweet and savory pulled pork is a reminder of summer that you can eat year round. It's also made in a slow cooker, so it's the perfect time-saving meal. Baked sweet potatoes make a great base to serve the delicious pulled pork on.

6 medium sweet potatoes, scrubbed with skins left on

3 lbs pork butt or picnic roast

2 tsp BBQ rub

3 cloves garlic

1 small onion, minced

½ cup brewed coffee

2 tsp cider vinegar

1 cup water or beer

1. Rub BBQ seasoning all over pork roast and place in slow cooker or crockpot.
2. Add remaining ingredients except sweet potatoes and set on med to low heat for 8 hours. Pork will shred easily with a fork when done.
3. When pork is nearly done, wrap 6 sweet potatoes in foil and bake at 350° F for 1 hour or until soft.
4. Split potatoes and top each with ⅔ cup of the shredded pork.

Calories 690 | Carbs 19g | Fat 40g | Protein 55g

HOW TO USE IT IN YOUR SWEET POTATO CYCLE

This meal serves as 1 serving of carbs, about 3-4 servings of fat, and 1 serving of protein. This one is so calorically dense and so good, you can use it as a reward meal.

NOTE: If you grab and use a sweet potato the size of your fist, you can be sure it's one serving of carbs.

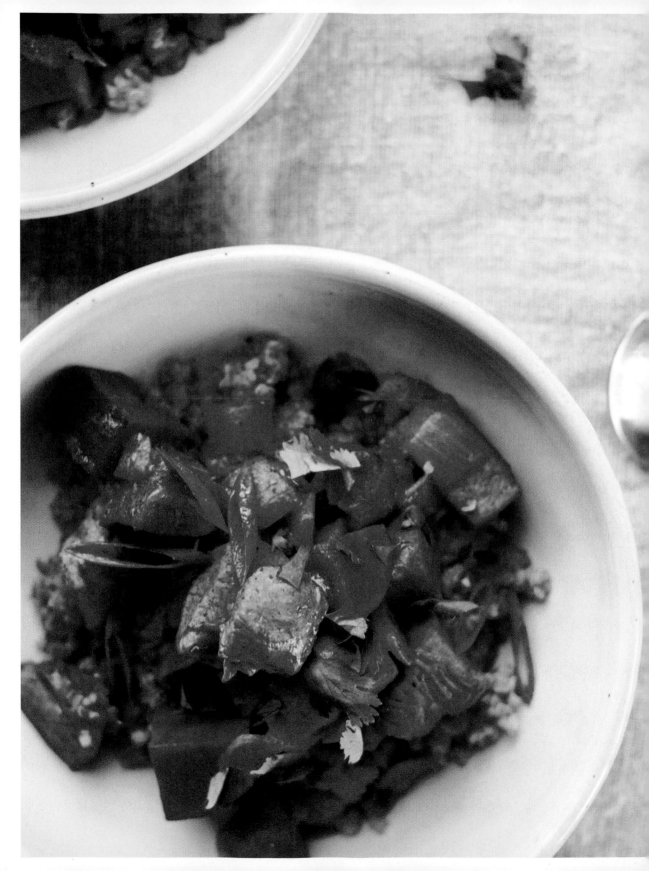

Chicken Sweet Potato Curry

Prep time: 15 minutes | Cook time: 20 minutes | Serves 4

Curry is a great way to add a different flavor to a sweet potato dish. The powerhouse, nutrient-rich garlic is a perfect pairing with curry powder and the sweet potato itself.

1 lb boneless chicken thigh or breast, cubed

1 small sweet potato, cubed or spiraled

1 small onion, chopped

1 clove garlic

1 can coconut milk

1 tbsp curry powder

1. In a large skillet, brown the chicken.
2. Add onions and cook until translucent. Add garlic and cook for another minute, then add curry powder and cook another minute to let the flavors develop.
3. Next, add one can of coconut milk. Refill the can with water, and add that as well.
4. Now, add the sweet potatoes. Turn the heat down to low and let cook until sweet potatoes are tender.
5. Serve over quinoa or rice.

Calories 292 | Carbs 16g | Fat 13g | Protein 29g

HOW TO USE IT IN YOUR SWEET POTATO CYCLE

This meal serves as 1 serving of carbs, a serving of fat, and a serving of protein (maybe a little more). Again, don't worry about consuming more protein.

*NOTE: *If you grab and use a sweet potato the size of your fist, you can be sure it's one serving of carbs.*

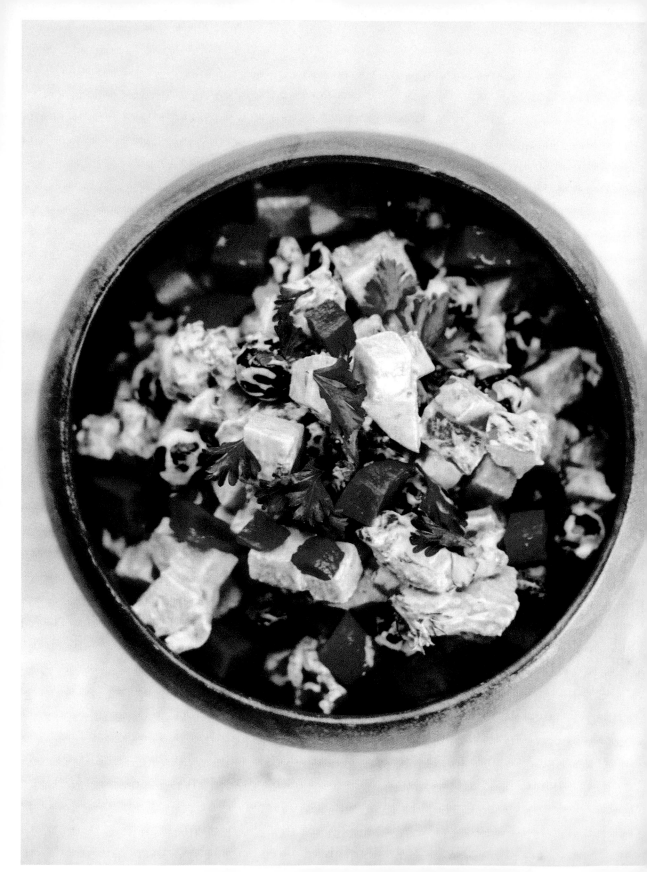

Chicken Salad

Prep time: 20 minutes | Cook time: 2 minutes | Serves 4

Chicken salad is really a great warm-weather option for those looking for a cool snack. Use the chicken salad as the main course in lettuce wraps or even as a fun party dip for carrot chips and celery! Plump fruits add just enough sweetness to this savory chicken dish.

1 lb cooked chicken breast	½ cup Greek yogurt (fat-free)
1 small sweet potato, cubed	¼ cup parsley, chopped
1 small apple, chopped	1 clove garlic, minced
½ cup grapes	1 tsp salt
¼ cup walnuts, chopped	1 tbsp apple cider vinegar

1. Microwave the cubed sweet potatoes in a dish for 2 minutes and then let cool.
2. Mix remaining ingredients in a bowl.
3. Once sweet potato is cool, add that to the bowl as well.
4. Refrigerate until ready to eat.

Calories 326 | Carbs 18g | Fat 12g | Protein 27g

HOW TO USE IT IN YOUR SWEET POTATO CYCLE

This meal serves as 1 serving of carbs, a serving of fat, and a healthy serving of protein. Again, don't worry about consuming more protein. I don't want you to worry about protein or veggies.

*NOTE: *If you grab and use a sweet potato the size of your fist, you can be sure it's one serving of carbs.*

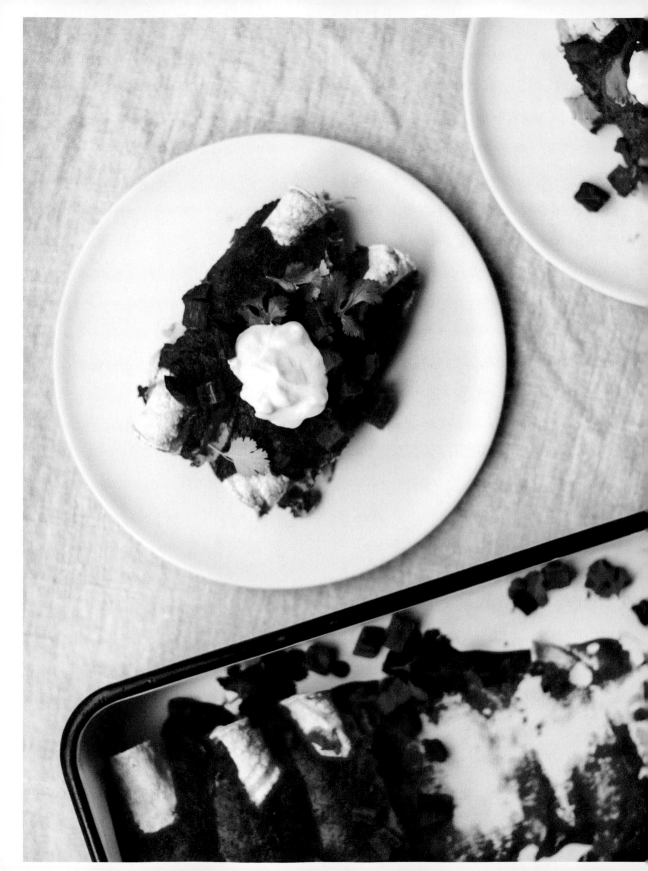

Enchiladas

Prep time: 15 minutes | Cook time: 30 minutes | Serves 6

Enchiladas are a hot and delicious way to enjoy Mexican food. Serve hot and top with the creamy enchilada sauce to make this meal perfect. The sweet potato inside is the perfect complement to this traditional dish.

FILLING

2 cups shredded cooked chicken

2 medium sweet potatoes, cooked and cubed

SAUCE

1 can tomato sauce

1 8 oz jar roasted red peppers, drained

1 cup Greek yogurt (fat-free)

12 tortillas (use coconut or almond flour tortillas if possible)

1. Preheat oven to 350° F.
2. Microwave the cubed sweet potatoes in a dish for 2 minutes until soft.
3. Mix together the cubed potato and shredded chicken in a bowl.
4. Place the sauce ingredients in a blender and puree until smooth.
5. To assemble, spoon one quarter of the sauce into the bottom of a 9x13 baking dish. Fill each tortilla with ⅓ cup of the filling, roll up the tortilla, and arrange in the dish.
6. Pour the remaining sauce on top and bake until hot and bubbly, approximately 30 minutes.

Calories 277 | Carbs 36g | Fat 2g | Protein 25g

HOW TO USE IT IN YOUR SWEET POTATO CYCLE

This meal serves as 1–2 servings of carbs and a serving of protein.

***NOTE:** If you grab and use a sweet potato the size of your fist, you can be sure it's one serving of carbs.

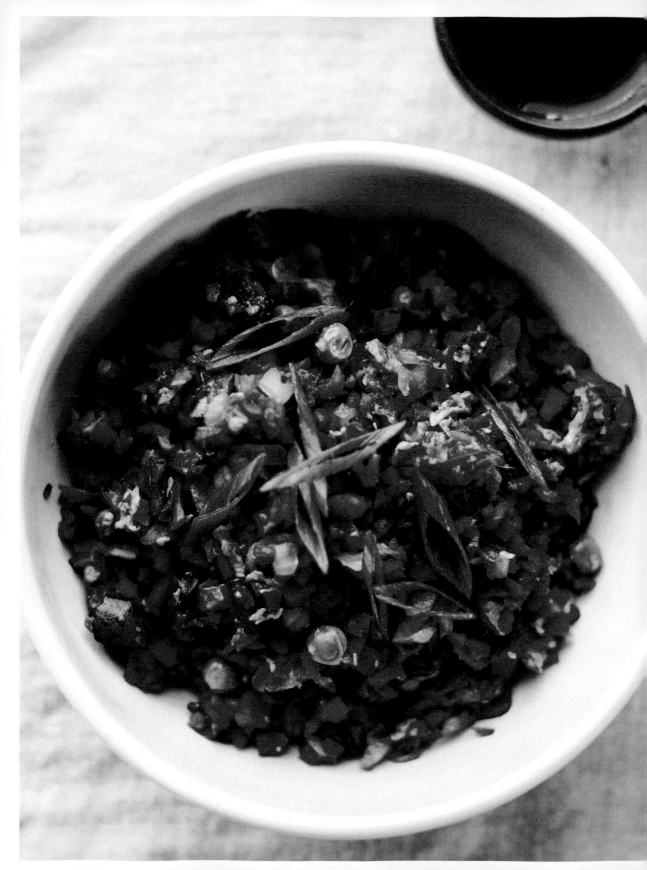

Fried Sweet Potato Rice

Prep time: 10 minutes | Cook time: 5 minutes | Serves 2

This recipe is a great breakfast or dinner dish. The best way to save time with this dish is to chop the ingredients ahead of time. The ginger gives an added warmth to the rich-sweet potato.

1 medium sweet potato

1 small onion, chopped

½ cup peas

3 small mushrooms, chopped

1 clove garlic, microplaned

½ inch piece of ginger, microplaned

"soy" sauce (Bragg or coconut liquid aminos)

2 eggs, beaten

1. Quarter the sweet potato and place in food processor. Pulse until it has a "rice" look to it.
2. Spray coconut oil in a skillet and add the sweet potato. Cook for just a few minutes and add the onion. Stir another few minutes, then add the garlic, ginger, peas, and mushrooms.
3. Let all of that cook down for a few more minutes, then drizzle the liquid aminos over everything. Push all of that to the side and add the eggs. Gently swirl the eggs as they cook and then slowly start to stir the rest of the pan into the eggs. Once the eggs are no longer wiggly it's done.

Calories 254 | Carbs 34g | Fat 8g | Protein 14g

HOW TO USE IT IN YOUR SWEET POTATO CYCLE

This meal serves as 1-2 servings of carbs, a little less than a serving of fat, and three-fourths of a serving of protein.

***NOTE:** If you grab and use a sweet potato the size of your fist, you can be sure it's one serving of carbs.*

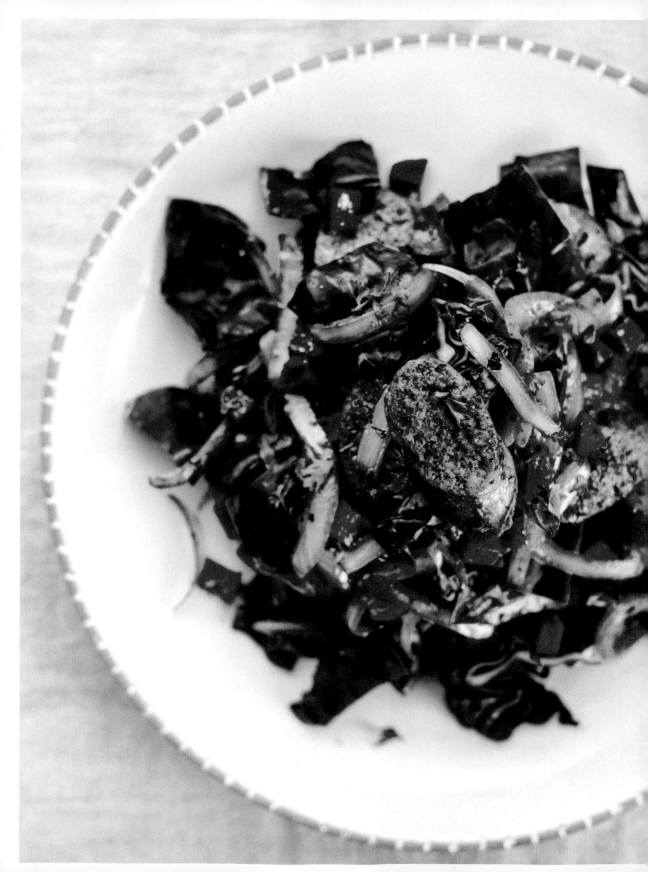

Kielbasa Sweet Potato and Cabbage

Prep time: 15 minutes | Cook time: 40 minutes | Serves 4–6

Kielbasa is a delicious pairing with the sweet potatoes in this traditional cabbage dish. Use your favorite spicy mustard to add a kick of flavor to this recipe.

1 lb organic sausage, sliced

½ onion, sliced

2 small sweet potatoes, peeled and cubed

½ small head of cabbage, 1½" slices then cubed

½ cup apple cider

1 tbsp spicy mustard

½ tsp dried basil

salt and pepper

1. In a large skillet, add olive oil and brown sausage. Add onion, sweet potato, and cabbage, pour in apple cider, mustard, basil, salt, and pepper.
2. Cover and let simmer 30 minutes.

Calories 346 | Carbs 34g | Fat 11g | Protein 21g

HOW TO USE IT IN YOUR SWEET POTATO CYCLE

This meal serves as 1½-2 servings of carbs, a serving of fat, and a serving of protein.

NOTE: If you grab and use a sweet potato the size of your fist, you can be sure it's one serving of carbs

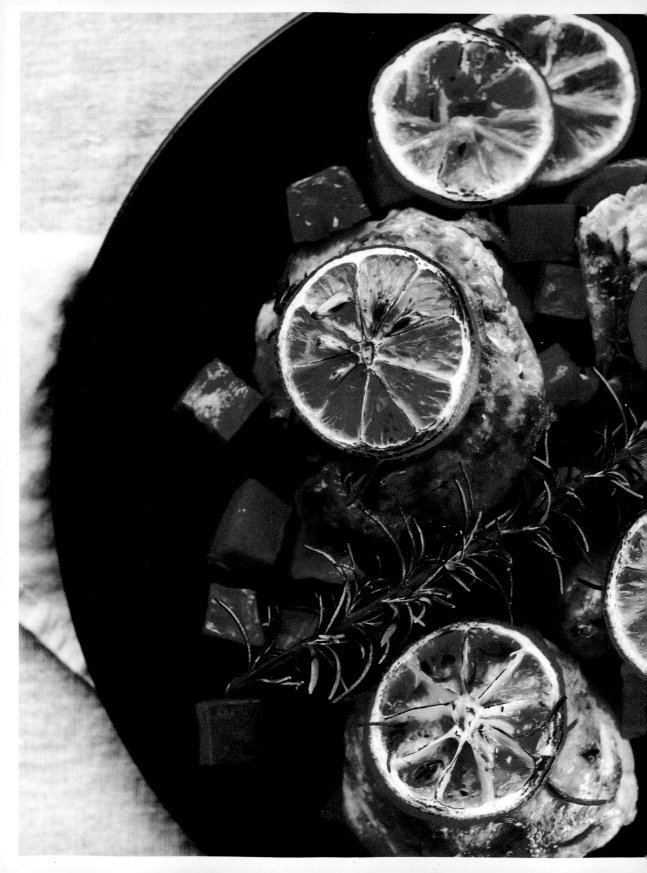

Lemon Garlic Sweet Potato Chicken

Prep time: 10 minutes | Cook time: 30 minutes | Serves 2

Lemon and garlic is a simple yet vibrant and delicious combination that not only makes the chicken thighs pop with flavor, but also complements the sweet potato. This dish is sure to be a simple-to-prepare family favorite.

4 chicken thighs

1 large sweet potato, cubed

1 lemon

3 cloves garlic

½ tsp salt

½ tsp pepper

coconut oil spray

1. Preheat oven to 400° F.
2. Place chicken, potatoes, and garlic cloves in a baking pan. Squeeze lemon juice over chicken, potatoes, and garlic.
3. Sprinkle with salt and pepper.
4. Bake for 30 minutes or until chicken reaches 165° F.

Calories 264 | Carbs 17g | Fat 10g | Protein 27g

HOW TO USE IT IN YOUR SWEET POTATO CYCLE

This meal serves as 1 serving of carbs, a serving of fat and a serving of protein (maybe a little more).

NOTE: *If you grab and use a sweet potato the size of your fist, you can be sure it's one serving of carbs.*

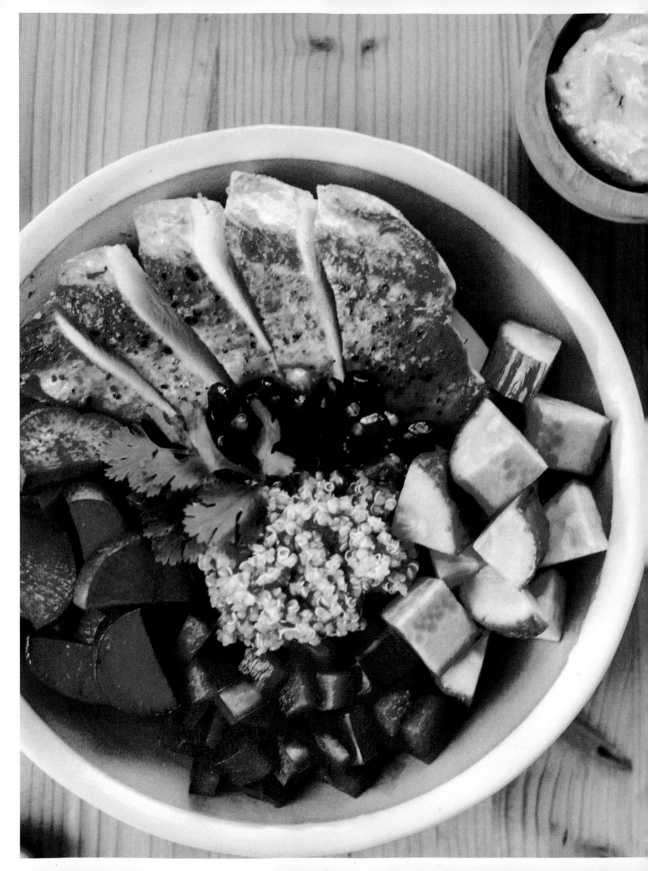

Roast Sweet Potato Salad Bowl

Prep time: 20 minutes | Cook time: 25 minutes | Serves 4

Between the chicken breast and the quinoa, this protein-rich salad bowl is sure to keep you full. Pomegranate keeps the flavor light and bright, and the dressing is so good, you will want to make it for your other salads.

2 small sweet potatoes, cut in half lengthwise and sliced

1 tsp olive oil

salt and pepper to taste

8 oz cooked and sliced chicken breast

½ cup diced yellow or red bell pepper

½ cup sliced cucumber

1 cup cooked quinoa

¼ cup pomegranate seeds

FOR THE DRESSING:

1 avocado

½ cup Greek yogurt (fat-free)

2 tbsp lemon juice

2 tbsp minced cilantro

1 clove garlic

pinch of salt

1. Preheat oven to 400° F. Toss potatoes with olive oil, salt, and pepper.
2. Roast sweet potatoes for 25 minutes, until tender. Cool to room temperature.
3. In a blender, add all of the dressing ingredients and blend for 30 seconds, until smooth. Thin with a bit of water to get desired consistency.
4. Assemble salad by arranging potatoes, sliced chicken, cucumber, and peppers around the sides of a bowl.
5. Heap quinoa in the center and scatter pomegranate seeds across the top. Drizzle with dressing.

Calories 386 | Carbs 43g | Fat 13g | Protein 23g

HOW TO USE IT IN YOUR SWEET POTATO CYCLE

This meal serves as 2–2½ serving of carbs, a serving of fat, and a serving a protein (maybe a little less). This is a good dish to which you can add some additional protein.

***NOTE:** If you grab and use a sweet potato the size of your fist, you can be sure it's one serving of carbs.*

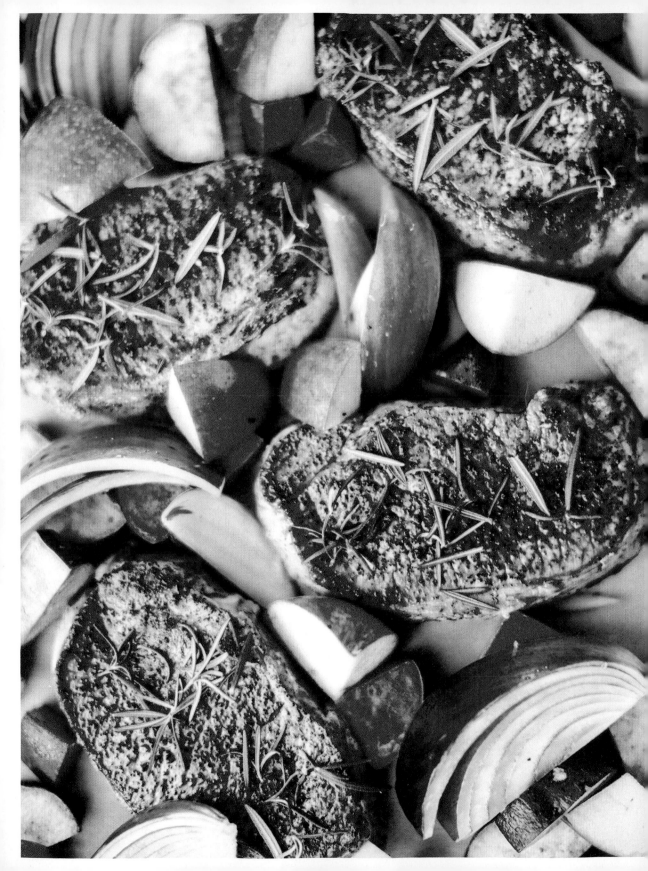

Rustic Pork Chops

Prep time: 10 minutes | Cook time: 45 minutes | Serves 4

These pork chops are sure to become a family favorite. Enjoy the crisp, sweet taste of the granny smith apples paired with sweet potatoes, with just a hint of rosemary to round out these vibrant flavors.

4 thick-cut pork chops

1 Granny Smith apple, chopped into big chunks

½ red onion, chopped into big chunks

2 small sweet potatoes, skin on, chopped into big chunks

salt and pepper

2 sprigs fresh rosemary

1. Preheat oven to 375° F.
2. Spray roasting pan or baking dish with coconut oil.
3. Place all ingredients in the pan. Cover with foil.
4. Cook 30 minutes covered and then 13 minutes uncovered.

Calories 470 | Carbs 23g | Fat 22g | Protein 28g

HOW TO USE IT IN YOUR SWEET POTATO CYCLE

This meal serves as about 1 serving of carbs, two servings of fat, and a serving of protein (maybe a little more).

*NOTE: *If you grab and use a sweet potato the size of your fist, you can be sure it's one serving of carbs.*

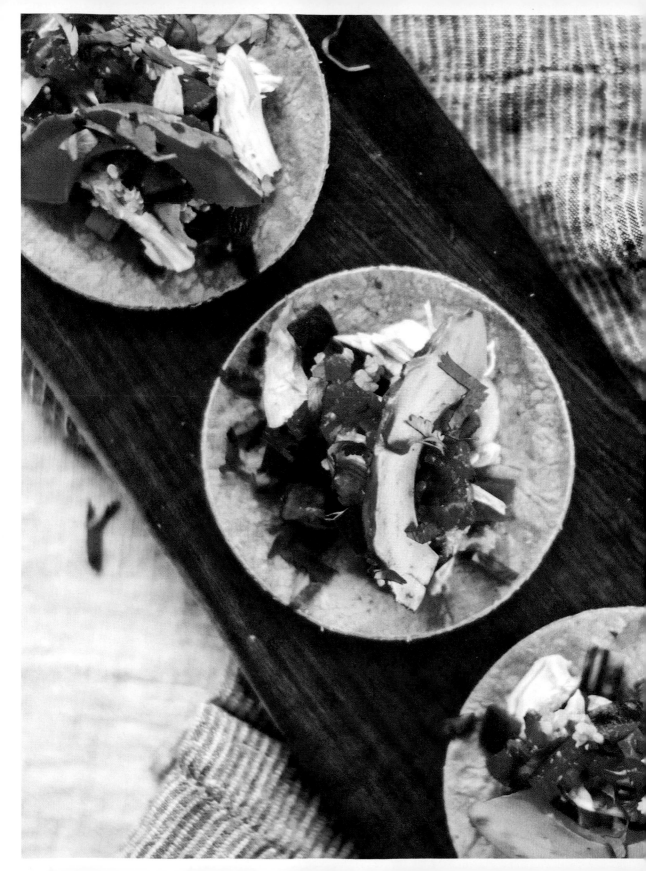

Salsa Verde Chicken and Sweet Potato Tacos

Prep time: 30 minutes | Cook time: 30 minutes | Serves 6

Who doesn't love tacos? Especially tacos with chicken and sweet potatoes! This dish is just perfect, and easy to make, too. Enjoy this dish and top with your favorite taco vegetable toppings and hot sauce or salsa.

1 lb chicken breast

salsa verde (you can make your own with

  the recipe below, or you can use jarred salsa)

1 large sweet potato, cubed

1 cup cooked quinoa

1 avocado, chopped

1 red pepper, chopped

tortillas

1. Preheat oven to 400° F.
2. Place chicken in a roasting pan and pour the salsa verde over it. Place sweet potatoes around the chicken.
3. Cover with foil and bake for 30 minutes or until chicken reaches 165° F.
4. You can shred the chicken then build your tacos using the quinoa, avocado, and red pepper.

SALSA VERDE

4 or 5 medium tomatillos, husked and washed

1 small onion

1 jalapeno, seeded

½ cup cilantro

Just one step: Everything goes in a food processor. Process until combined.

Calories 282 | Carbs 25g | Fat 8g | Protein 27g

HOW TO USE IT IN YOUR SWEET POTATO CYCLE

This meal serves as 1 serving of carbs (maybe a little more), a little less than 1 serving of fat, and a serving of protein (maybe a little more).

NOTE: If you grab and use a sweet potato the size of your fist, you can be sure it's one serving of carbs.

Shepherd's Pie

Prep time: 25 minutes | Cook time: 30 minutes | Serves 8

Our shepherd's pie only takes 30 minutes and makes for a great family dinner that will easily become the new favorite. This is a much healthier take on a classic dish.

PIE FILLING

1 lb ground beef

1 onion, chopped

1 clove garlic, chopped

2 carrots, chopped

1 tsp Italian seasoning

1 tbsp tomato paste

1 tbsp corn starch or potato starch

1 cup water

salt and pepper

MASHED SWEET POTATO

1 large sweet potato

½ cup Greek yogurt (fat free)

1 tsp salt

1. Preheat oven to 375° F.
2. Microwave sweet potato until tender (around 5 minutes).
3. While that cooks, brown beef with the onion, garlic, and carrots. Once browned, add potato starch and tomato paste, cook for a minute or two, then add Italian seasoning, salt and pepper, and water.
4. Cook another few minutes until thickened. Take off heat and prepare the mashed sweet potato topping.
5. Cut potato in half and scoop out filling.
6. Place potato filling in a bowl and add Greek yogurt and salt. Mash until fluffy.
7. Put beef mixture in a pie pan and top with mashed sweet potato. Bake for 30 minutes.

Calories 245 | Carbs 22g | Fat 10g | Protein 17g

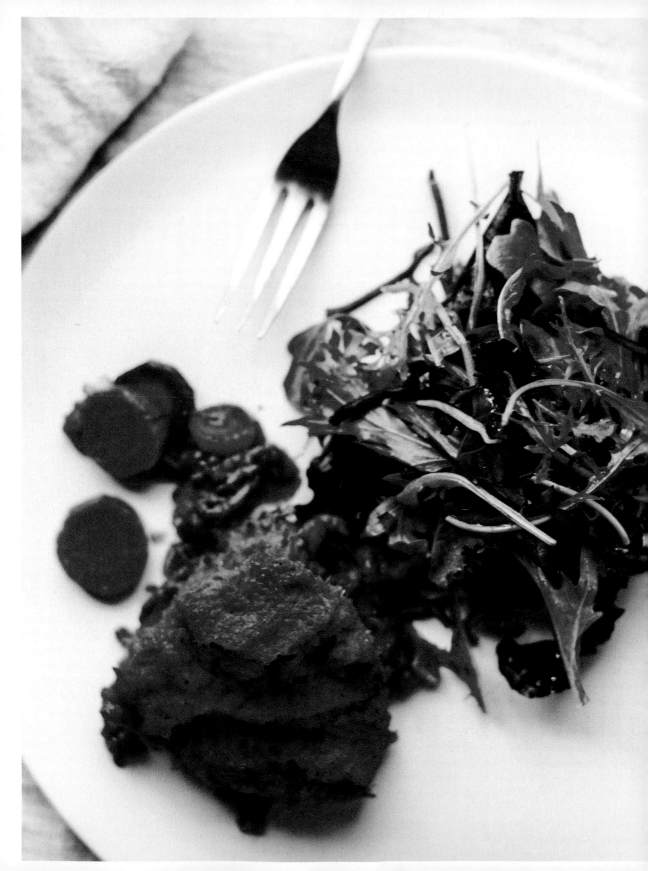

HOW TO USE IT IN YOUR SWEET POTATO CYCLE

This meal serves as 1 serving of carbs, a serving of fat, and a little less than one serving of protein (always varies based on the size of your palm).

*NOTE: *If you grab and use a sweet potato the size of your fist, you can be sure it's one serving of carbs.*

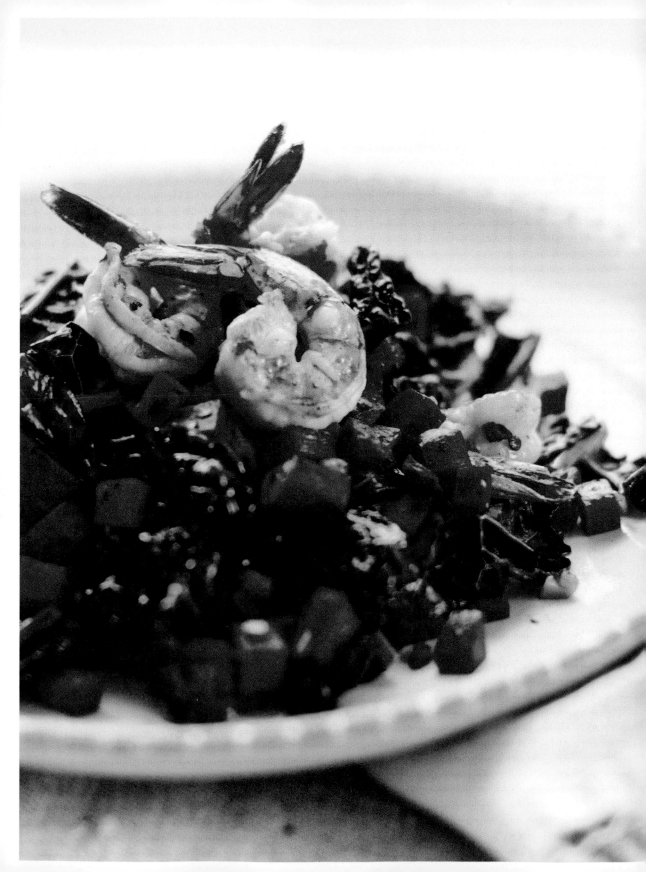

Shrimp, Sweet Potato, and Kale Sauté

Prep time: 15 minutes | Cook time: 20 minutes | Serves 2

This powerhouse dish is loaded with nutrients from the two super foods, kale and sweet potatoes. This dish cooks up quick and easy and can be light enough for a side, or eaten as an entire meal.

8 oz medium shrimp, raw, peeled, and deveined

1 large sweet potato, peeled and diced

2 cups kale, washed and chopped

1 tsp red pepper flakes

2 cloves garlic, minced

pinch of salt

2 tsp olive oil

1. Steam or boil diced sweet potato 15 minutes until partially cooked. Drain and set aside.
2. In a large sauté pan, heat olive oil over medium heat.
3. Add potato, pepper flakes, garlic, and salt. Sauté for 5 minutes, then add shrimp and kale.
4. Sauté 5 more minutes. Be careful not to overcook shrimp.

Calories 292 | Carbs 16g | Fat 13g | Protein 29g

HOW TO USE IT IN YOUR SWEET POTATO CYCLE

This meal serves as 1 serving of carbs (maybe a little less), a serving of fat, and a little more than a serving of protein (always varies based on the size of your palm).

***NOTE:** If you grab and use a sweet potato the size of your fist, you can be sure it's one serving of carbs.*

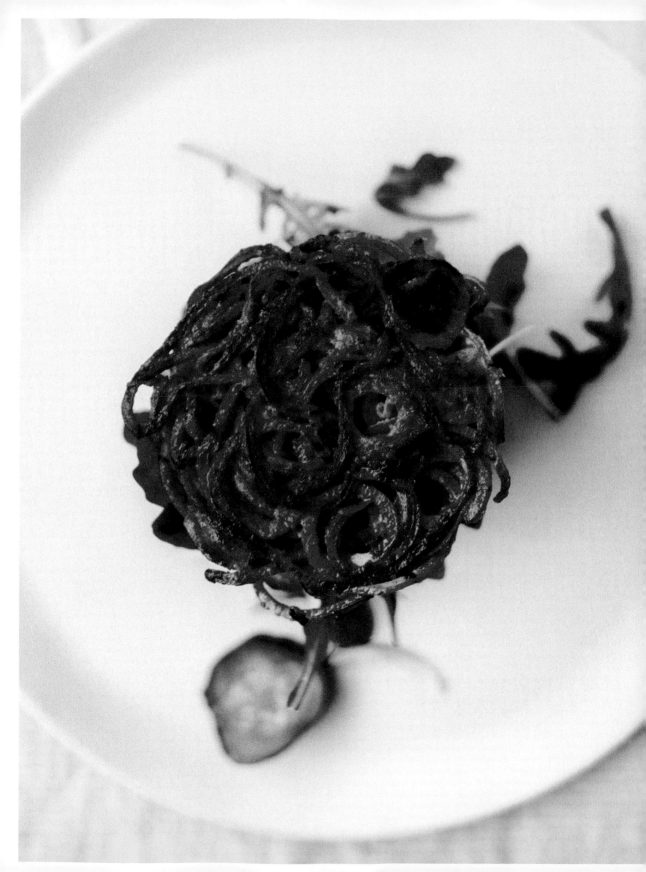

Spiraled Sweet Potato Bun

Prep time: 10 minutes | Cook time: 30 minutes | Serves 2 (makes 4 buns)

Who says you shouldn't play with your food? This spiraled sweet potato bun not only tastes great, but is a fun twist (pun intended) on your traditional bun. I first had these at a restaurant in Santa Monica and they were excellent. And now you can eat burgers with a bun that's good for you.

> 1 large sweet potato, spiraled
> 1 egg
> 1 tbsp coconut flour
> cayenne powder
> Coconut Oil

1. Mix the spiraled sweet potato with the egg, flour, and seasoning.
2. Using a hamburger press (or your hands) shape the buns.
3. Heat coconut oil in a skillet over medium or medium-high heat.
4. Fry each patty until golden brown.

Calories 124 | Carbs 17g | Fat 4g | Protein 5g

HOW TO USE IT IN YOUR SWEET POTATO CYCLE

This meal serves as 1 serving of carbs (maybe a little less). Add some protein and turn it into a great meal; grass-fed beef or chicken.

NOTE: If you grab and use a sweet potato the size of your fist, you can be sure it's one serving of carbs.

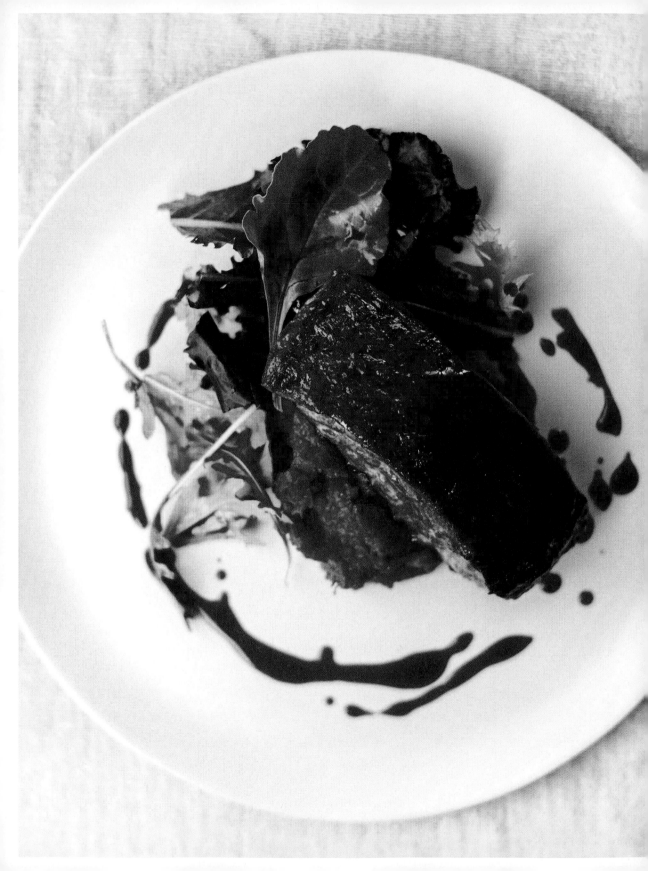

Sriracha Salmon and Ginger Sweet Potato

Prep time: 70 minutes | Cook time: 20 minutes | Serves 2

Salmon is a fantastic source of protein and omega-3 fatty acids. Combine your salmon with a side of sweet potatoes for an incredibly healthy dinner. This is one dish that tastes as amazing as it looks.

4 6 oz salmon fillets

¼ cup Sriracha

¼ cup honey

1 clove garlic, micro-planed

MASHED GINGER SWEET POTATO

2 medium sweet potatoes, microwaved

1 inch piece ginger, microplaned

1 tbsp butter

1. Mix the sriracha, honey, and garlic together, and place in a large ziploc bag with the salmon. Refrigerate for 1 hour.
2. Preheat oven to 375° F. Bake salmon for 20 minutes until it is just cooked through.
3. While the salmon is baking, microwave the potatoes for 5-6 minutes, then peel and mash with ginger and butter.
4. Serve the salmon on top of the mashed potatoes.

Calories 547 | Carbs 50g | Fat 18g | Protein 44g

HOW TO USE IT IN YOUR SWEET POTATO CYCLE

This meal serves as 2 servings of carbs, 2 servings of fat, and a little more than a serving of protein (always varies based on the size of your palm).

*****NOTE:** *If you grab and use a sweet potato the size of your fist, you can be sure it's one serving of carbs.*

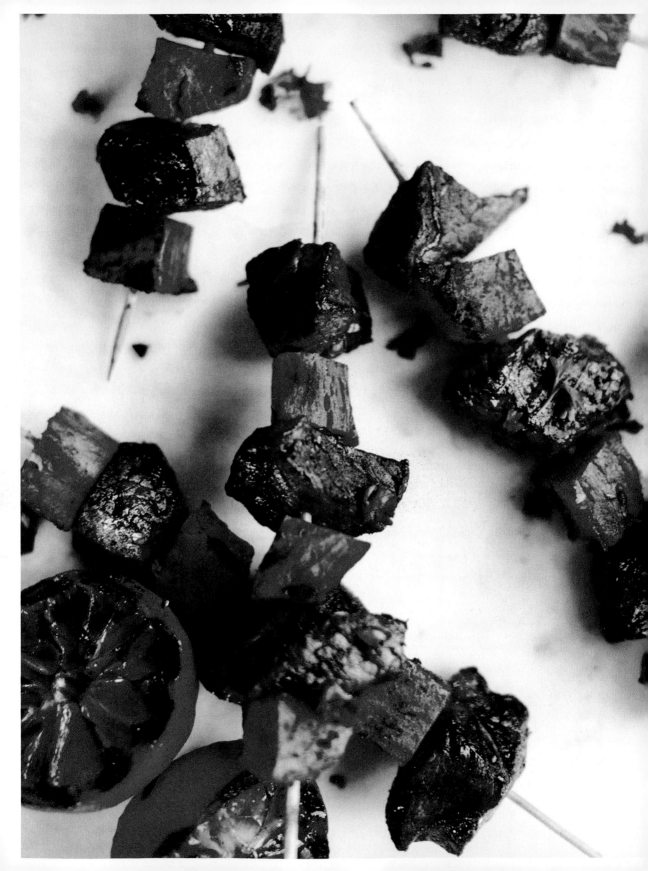

Steak Kabobs

Prep time: 70 minutes | Cook time: 15 minutes | Serves 2

If you're grilling, kabobs are a go-to dish that is fun, easy, and really tasty! Although they are also great baked in the oven, when cooked over the grill, the fire brings out a nice smoky flavor from the marinated steak and cubes of sweet potato.

16 oz sirloin steak, cubed into 1 inch pieces

1 large sweet potato

MARINADE

2 tbsp olive oil

3 tbsp balsamic vinegar

2 cloves garlic, minced

½ tsp dried oregano

½ tsp salt

1. Mix all ingredients of the marinade. Marinate the steak at least one hour, but preferably overnight.
2. Cook the potato 4 minutes in the microwave until about halfway cooked, then peel and cube into 1 inch pieces.
3. Fill skewers alternating between meat and sweet potatoes, then grill or bake until steak is at desired doneness. This should take about 10 minutes total for medium rare.

Calories 769 | Carbs 32g | Fat 39g | Protein 73g

HOW TO USE IT IN YOUR SWEET POTATO CYCLE

This meal serves as 1½–2 servings of carbs, 3–4 servings of fat, and about 2 servings of protein.

NOTE: If you grab and use a sweet potato the size of your fist, you can be sure it's one serving of carbs.

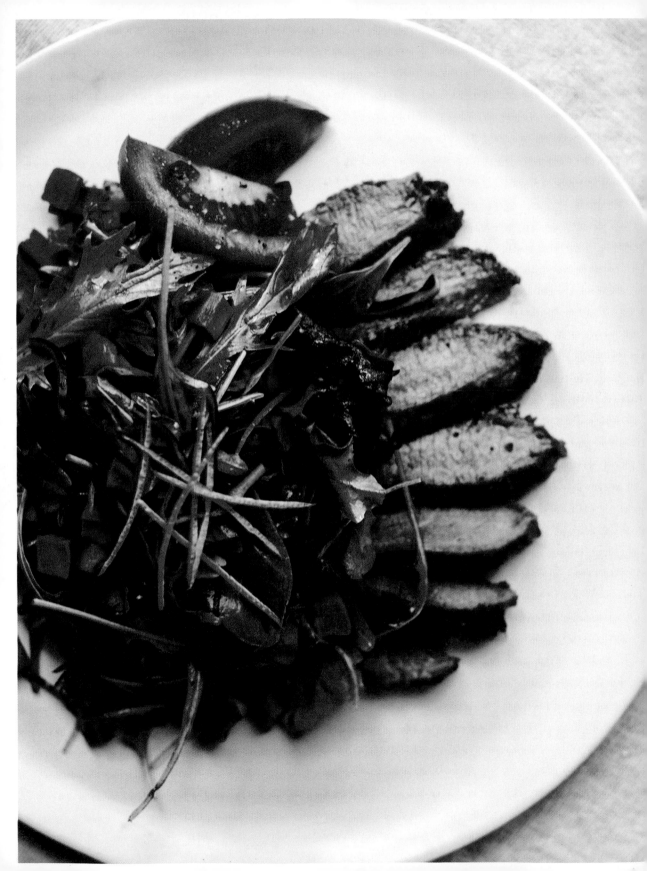

Steak Salad with Roasted Sweet Potato

Prep time: 10 minutes | Cook time: 5–10 minutes | Serves 2

This is a great take on steak and potatoes and is very easy to make. Great recipe to use if you have leftover steak. With just a couple ounces of steak, thinly sliced, you can make a healthy steak and sweet potato salad. Yum!

1–2 oz grilled steak, thinly sliced

1 cup roasted sweet potato cubes

Handful of mixed lettuce

Dressing: drizzle with oil and vinegar

1. Grill steak to desired temperature.
2. Preheat Oven to 425° F.
3. Toss cubed sweet potatoes with coconut oil or olive oil, and bake until fork tender.

Calories 202 | Carbs 39g | Fat 1g | Protein 10g

HOW TO USE IT IN YOUR SWEET POTATO CYCLE

This meal serves as 1½–2 servings of carbs, and about a ½ serving of protein.

*NOTE: If you grab and use a sweet potato the size of your fist, you can be sure it's one serving of carbs.

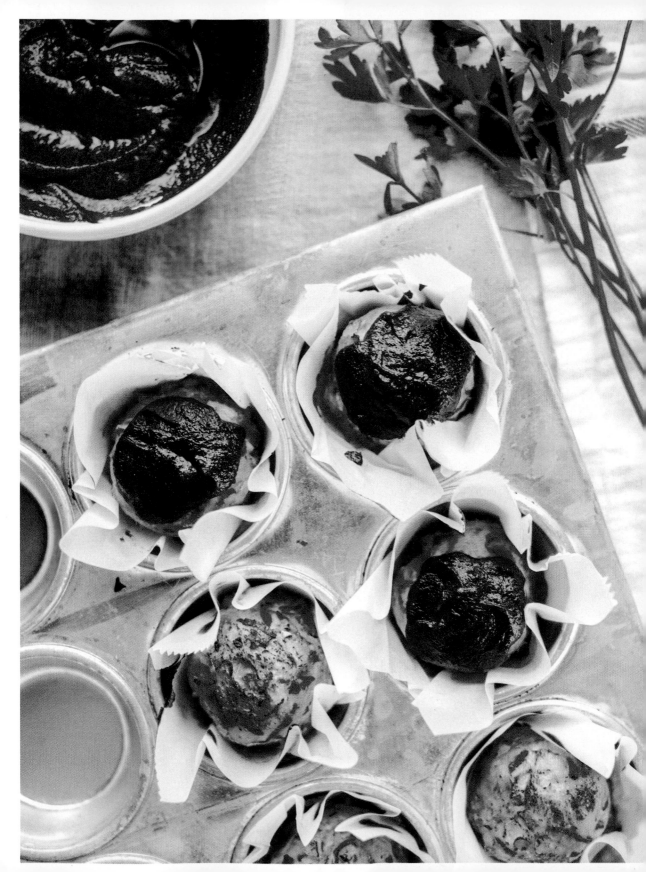

Turkey Loaf

Prep time: 10 minutes | Cook time: 20 minutes | Serves 6

Meatloaf is a staple. In fact, we eat it once a week. This truly loaf is insane, not to mention lean and healthy. Now the entire famlly can enjoy it.

TURKEY LOAF

1 lb ground turkey

½ cup sweet potato, shredded

¼ cup almond flour

¼ cup onion, chopped

2 cloves garlic, minced

¼ tsp salt

1 tsp Italian seasoning

SAUCE

¼ cup ketchup

1 tsp curry powder

1. Preheat oven to 375° F.
2. Mix all ingredients for turkey loaf, then form into balls.
3. Place in greased muffin tin and bake for 20 minutes.
4. Mix ketchup and curry powder together and top cooked turkey loaf muffins.

Calories 195 | Carbs 4g | Fat 10g | Protein 22g

HOW TO USE IT IN YOUR SWEET POTATO CYCLE

This meal serves as 1 serving of fat and 1 serving of protein.

NOTE: *If you grab and use a sweet potato the size of your fist, you can be sure it's one serving of carbs.*

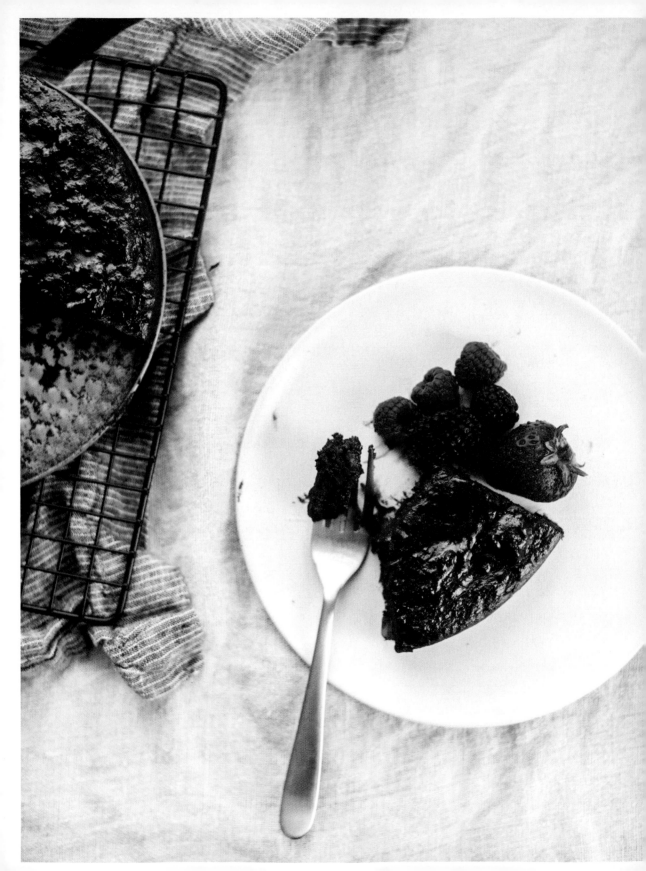

CHAPTER 15

Desserts: 6 Recipes

Sweet potatoes make desserts even better, not to mention healthier. Their sweet flavor and versatility in baking leave no question as to why they make a perfect sweet treat. Because these treats are so delicious, these are great desserts to have along with your reward meal, creating the perfect alternative to unhealthy cakes and pastries. When you use these desserts on your reward meal you really set yourself up for major success. Feel free to use them on your high-carb days, just plug them in as indicated below the recipe.

Keep something in mind with all of the desserts: I have overestimated the servings to take into account the sugar (natural of course, but still sugar). You can swap these on your high-carb days without missing a beat. How much do you love me now?

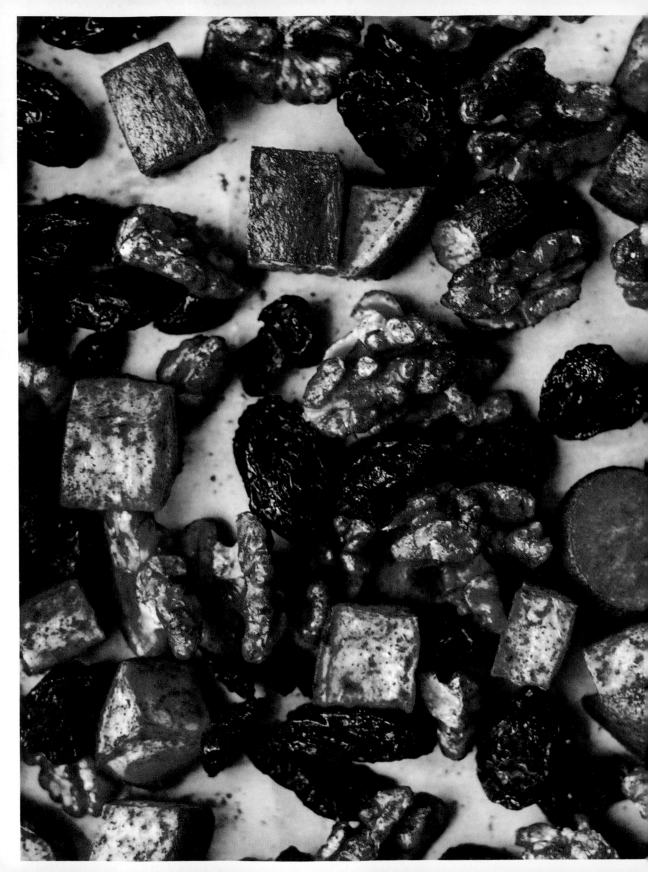

Candied Sweet Potato Bites

Prep time: 10 minutes | Cook time: 20 minutes | Serves 2

These sweet, bite-sized treats are perfect for stopping a sweet tooth dead in its tracks. The walnuts are very satiating, and the maple syrup and sweet potato combo hit the sweet notes—so good, they're going to be hard to share.

  1 smaller sweet potato, cubed

  ¼ cup raisins

  ¼ cup walnuts

  1 tsp cinnamon

  1 tbsp maple syrup

1. Preheat oven to 400° F.
2. Mix all ingredients and spread out on a parchment-lined baking sheet.
3. Cook for 20 minutes or until sweet potatoes are soft.

Calories 239 | Carbs 32g | Fat 10g | Protein 5g

HOW TO USE IT IN YOUR SWEET POTATO CYCLE

This meal serves as 2 servings of carbs (a little high here because of the glycemic load), 1 serving of fat, and not enough protein to count.

***NOTE:** If you grab and use a sweet potato the size of your fist, you can be sure it's one serving of carbs.*

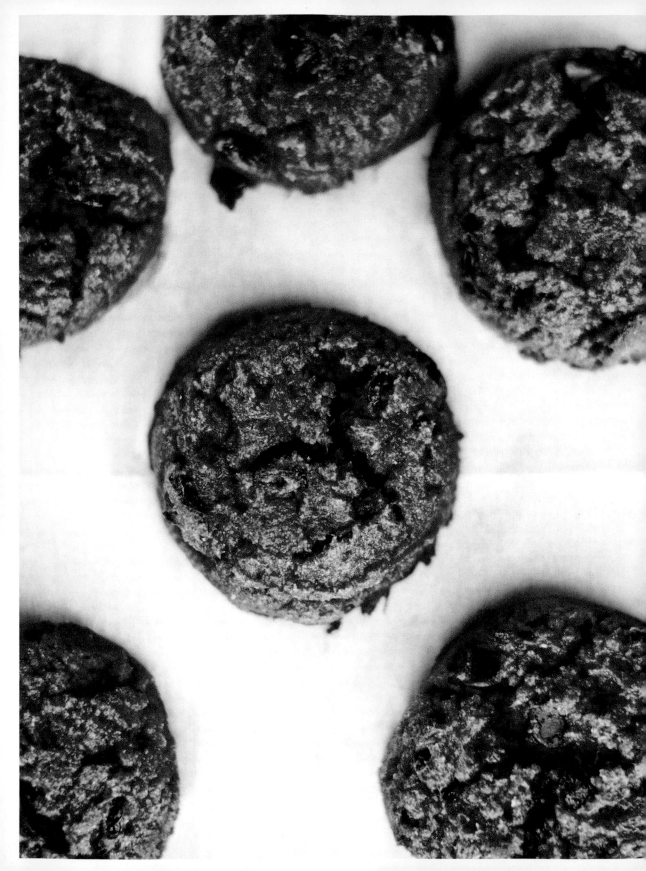

Chocolate Chip Sweet Potato Cookies

Prep time: 15 minutes | Cook time: 30 minutes | Makes 24 cookies

Chocolate chip cookies are the sweetheart of all desserts. These pair well with almond milk and can be dunked like a regular cookie, without all of the guilt. The sweet potato makes this snack filling and satisfying for those craving a little chocolate, as well.

1 egg

1 cup mashed sweet potato

¼ cup coconut milk

½ cup maple syrup

1 tsp vanilla

¼ cup coconut flour

¾ cup almond flour

1 tsp baking soda

1 tsp cinnamon

1 cup dried fruit

(raisins, cranberries, or cherries)

1. Preheat oven to 350° F.
2. Mix egg, sweet potato, coconut milk, maple syrup, and vanilla in a mixer until blended.
3. Add flours, baking soda, cinnamon, and fruit, and mix until combined.
4. Line a cookie sheet with parchment paper and drop cookies using a cookie scoop or spoon. These cookies do not spread, so pat them down flat if you do not want round cookies. Bake each batch for 13 minutes or until lightly browned on top.

Calories 71 | Carbs 11g | Fat 3g | Protein .5g

HOW TO USE IT IN YOUR SWEET POTATO CYCLE

This meal serves as ½–1 serving of carbs (factoring in a bit high because of the glycemic load in the fruit and syrup), and ½ serving of fat.

NOTE: If you grab and use a sweet potato the size of your fist, you can be sure it's one serving of carbs.

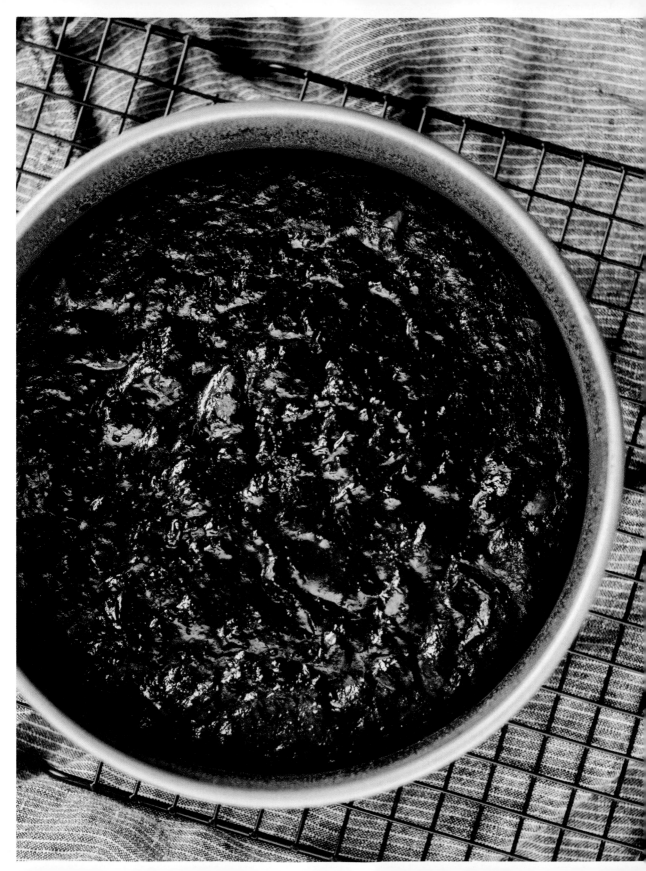

Chocolate Torte

Prep time: 20 minutes | Cook time: 20 minutes | Serves 8

They say you can't have your cake and eat it too, but that's just not true all of the time. I find ways to make my favorite desserts healthy so I can indulge from time to time. Ok, more than occasionally. I eat sweet things (healthy versions only) every week. I just build them into my cycle like you can here.

   This chocolate power house boasts a thick, yet creamy cake along with crunchy nuts and it will have you saying—oh, damn! You won't believe it's healthy.

   12 oz dark chocolate

   1½ cup mashed sweet potatoes

   ½ cup macadamia nuts, chopped

   3 eggs

   ½ tsp vanilla

   pinch of salt

1. Preheat oven to 350° F.
2. Microwave potatoes until soft, about 10 minutes. Scoop out flesh and mash.
3. Mix in chocolate, nuts, vanilla, and salt.
4. Once cooled, add eggs.
5. Pour into a 9-inch pie plate or square baking dish. Bake for 20 minutes.

Calories 215 | Carbs 18g | Fat 11g | Protein .5g

HOW TO USE IT IN YOUR SWEET POTATO CYCLE

This meal serves as 1½–2 servings of carbs, 1 serving of fat, and don't count the protein (it's not substantiated).

*NOTE: *If you grab and use a sweet potato the size of your fist, you can be sure it's one serving of carbs.*

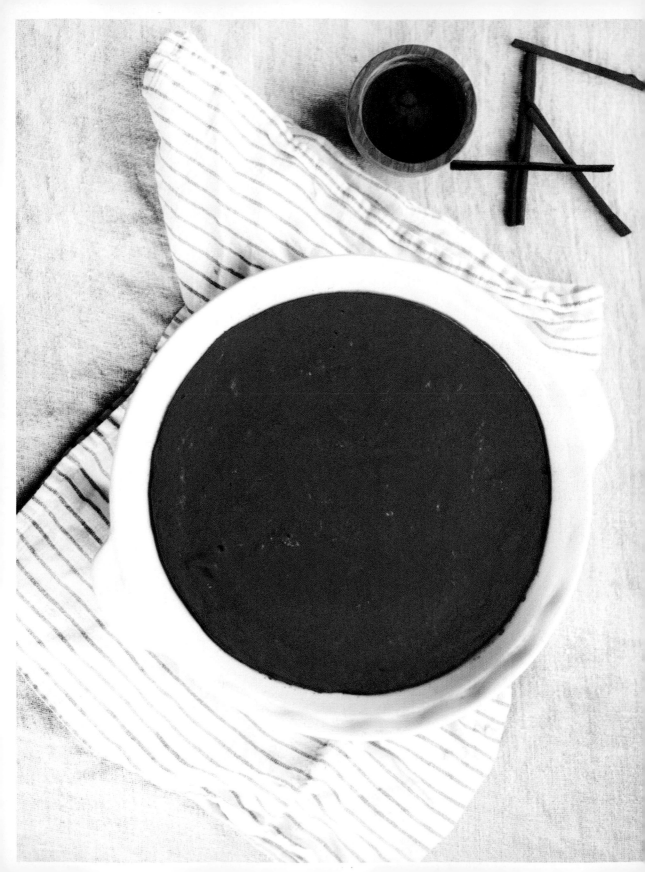

Crustless Sweet Potato Pie

Prep time: 40 minutes | Cook time: 30 minutes | Serves 8

You don't have to wait for Thanksgiving to enjoy this sweet potato pie. At least I don't! This recipe cuts out the crust, so you enjoy what you really came for, the goods. The sweet potatoes make an enjoyable pie for all those who enjoy traditional holiday treats on non-holidays.

1 large sweet potato, boiled until tender	3 eggs
½ cup butter	1 tsp vanilla
¼ cup maple syrup	½ tsp cinnamon
pinch of salt	¼ tsp nutmeg

1. In a pot, bring water to a boil, and place in sweet potato.
2. Once tender, take out sweet potato and mash.
3. In a large bowl add in the remaining ingredients and mix until thoroughly combined.
4. Preheat oven to 350° F.
5. Spray pie plate with coconut oil.
6. Spread batter in pan and bake for 30 minutes.

Calories 179 | Carbs 10g | Fat 14g | Protein 3g

HOW TO USE IT IN YOUR SWEET POTATO CYCLE

This meal serves as 1 serving of carbs and 1–2 servings of fat.

NOTE: If you grab and use a sweet potato the size of your fist, you can be sure it's one serving of carbs.

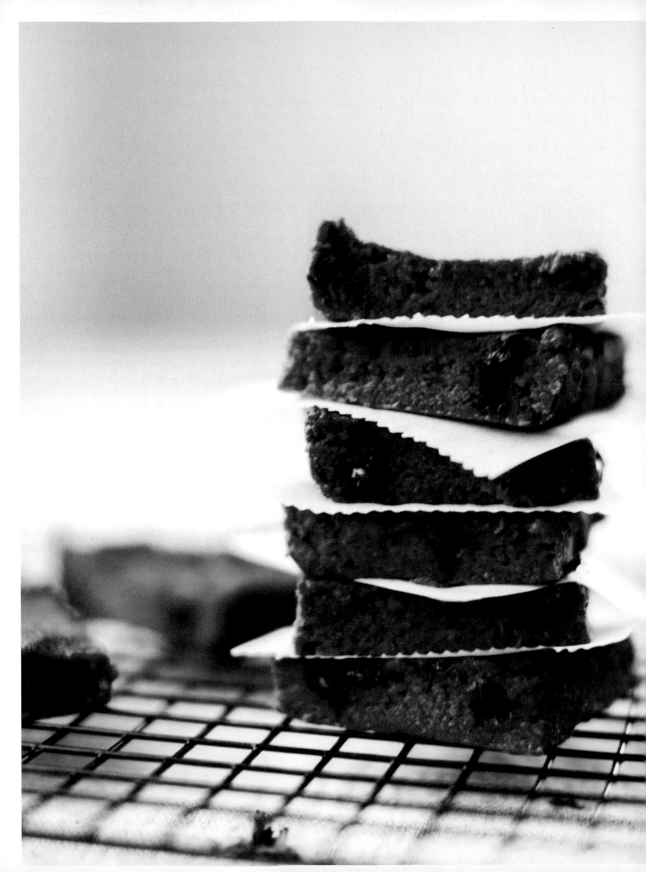

Sweet Potato Brownies

Prep time: 15 minutes | Cook time: 20 minutes | Serves 12 (depending on cut size)

Brownies are one of my favorites! An easy, go-to sweet. I am not sure I even know one person that doesn't like brownies. If you were following me on Snapchat, you'd know I have a dish of these in my refrigerator right now. Serious! They are the bomb. You can thank me later.

1 cup mashed sweet potato

2 eggs

½ cup honey

¼ cup coconut oil

1 tsp vanilla

½ cup coconut flour

⅓ cup cocoa powder

¼ tsp baking powder

¼ tsp salt

½ cup dark chocolate chips (optional)

1. Preheat oven to 350° F.
2. Lightly coat a 9x9 inch pan with coconut oil.
3. Mix the sweet potato, eggs, honey, coconut oil, and vanilla.
4. Add flour, cocoa powder, baking powder, and salt (and chocolate chips, if using).
5. Mix gently until combined. Pour into greased 9x9 inch pan and bake for 20 minutes.
6. Brownies are done when you can insert a knife and it comes out clean.

Calories 181 | Carbs 24g | Fat 10g | Protein 3g

HOW TO USE IT IN YOUR SWEET POTATO CYCLE—

This meal serves as 2 servings of carbs and 1 serving of fat.

*__NOTE:__ *If you grab and use a sweet potato the size of your fist, you can be sure it's one serving of carbs.*

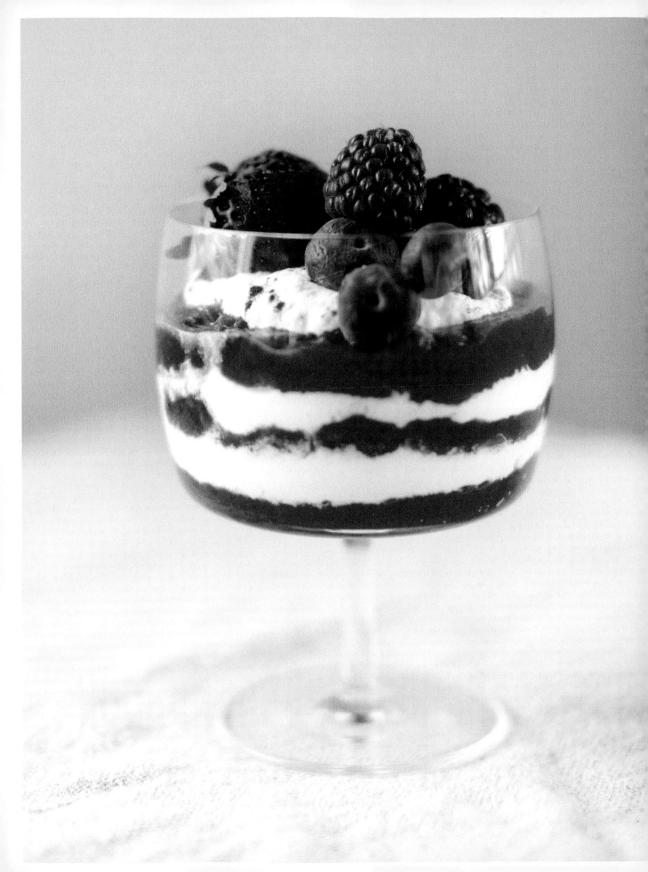

Sweet Potato Parfait

Prep time: 15 minutes | Cook time: 30 minutes | Serves 2

Each layer of this parfait is more delicious than the last. Bye-bye, traditional parfait! The spices keep your taste buds digging for more, and the sweet potatoes make this dessert a filling one!

1 medium sweet potato

2 tbsp maple syrup

1 tsp cinnamon

¼ tsp ground cardamom

1 cup Greek yogurt (fat free)

1 scoop vanilla Morellifit Nutrition Protein (link under section on supplementation)

1. Peel, quarter, and boil the sweet potato until tender. Drain and mash with maple syrup, cinnamon, and cardamom until smooth. Set aside and let cool.
2. Mix Greek yogurt and Morellifit Nutrition Protein, then alternate large spoonfuls of yogurt with spoonfuls of sweet potato in a glass.
3. You should have a total of 5 layers. Top with an additional sprinkle of cinnamon, if desired.

Calories 153 | Carbs 18g | Fat 2g | Protein 8.5g

HOW TO USE IT IN YOUR SWEET POTATO CYCLE

This meal serves as 2 servings of carbs and about ½ a serving of protein.

NOTE: If you grab and use a sweet potato the size of your fist, you can be sure it's one serving of carbs.

PART 4:

THE PATH TO LONG TERM HEALTH BENEFITS

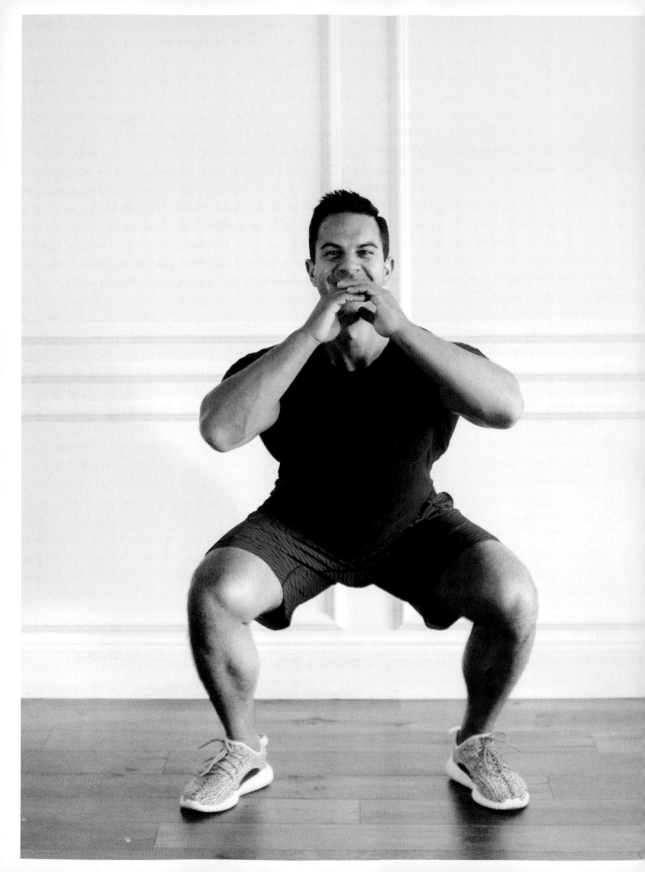

CHAPTER 16

Exercising Around Your Super Carb Cycle

I f you choose (which I hope you do) to exercise while on the Sweet Potato Diet, there are a few things you can do to get the most out of it. If you're unsure of where to start, below you'll find some really great short but effective training routines. Even if you've never exercised before in your life (or in years), they have been put together step-by-step so you can get going today. Whether you do the below routines, choose your favorite activity, or already go to the gym, the key to lasting health and long-term sustainability is exercise. Not too much exercise, just some, every day.

What If I've Never Really Trained Before?

I know workouts are probably the last thing on your mind, and that's OK. I promise to keep them short and sweet. You can even choose to walk around the block if you'd like. The key is to just stay active. Forget about long, rigorous workouts while you're on the Sweet Potato Diet (unless, of course, you're already in a routine).

This is a chapter for people who dislike working out or find it overly complicated and intimidating. Because I know you hate working out so much, I decided I would create a section specifically for you. I put together a workout plan that is done right from home with absolutely no equipment and only takes 3 minutes to complete (Yep. That's all you need right now). Let's let the Sweet Potato Diet do the heavy lifting.

This 3-minute workout is so simple, you cannot fail. In fact, if for whatever reason you do "fail," you don't keep pushing until you are comfortable. Maybe you're saying to yourself… "Michael, I thought you were legit and now I'm confused. You're telling me I can stop training?"

YES. But let me finish, please. Remember, my goal is to help you get to the next level and to build better habits, and I know, based on working with hundreds of thousands of clients, that if we go too fast, you will fail.

Not to mention, it's the diet I want you to focus on, not the training (I am not saying training isn't important either). I am just saying diet and nutrition make up over 80% plus of the fat loss equation.

After working with people in the fitness industry for so long, I've found a common denominator among everyone who trains every day. It is this: they didn't start out that way. I didn't start out training for 90 minute per day 6 days per week, and if I would have I would have failed. You see, I just didn't enjoy it like I do now.

The majority don't just magically become fitness buffs overnight. In fact, if you ask most people, they'll tell you that, at one point or another, they didn't even like working out at all.

Most built habits bit-by-bit over time, and that's exactly what we are going to do, starting with 3 minutes of training (not a minute more). I am asking you to just trust me on this. The gym is just a barrier right now if you're currently not regularly training. Remember, if you *are* currently training, just keep on doing your thing, and later in this chapter I will help you tweak your cycle to work in conjunction with your current training schedule to really maximize your results.

3 MINUTES—NOTHING MORE

Can you give me 3 minutes, first thing in the morning? I'm being totally serious. That's it. Three minutes is all I'm asking from you. And you can do that for as long as it takes for you to give me 3 minutes a day for 7 consecutive days.

In fact, that's your exercise goal number one.

Goal—Three minutes of exercise for 7 consecutive days.

If you do it in the first 7 days, then kudos to you. If it takes a few weeks to nail 7 consecutive days in a row, that's perfectly fine, too. I don't even care if it takes you several months; remember, diet is where the real magic happens.

The beauty of this process is that there is no timeline. There is no rush, and there is no need to be perfect. As you nail your workouts, you'll begin to rewire your brain. Remember, you're used to not training, and we need to reprogram your brain. We do that through simplification. That's how new habits are formed. We need to show your brain that you are in control. We love to be in control or at least to think we are. And when you choose to train for three minutes, guess what? Yep, you are in control. Now you're a control freak, haha!

The idea is, as you continue choosing to train for 3 minutes a day, it's only a matter of time before you choose to train for 4, 5, and so on. So, you've nailed 7 consecutive days at 3 minutes, can I ask that on day 8 you push just one more minute?

Can I have 4 minutes every morning beginning on day 8?

Now **you're on a roll!**

Nice work. How does it feel to be in control?

After you've nailed 4 minutes for 7 consecutive days, how about adding just one more minute? So on day 15, ramp up to 5 minutes (don't worry, the workouts are coming up). Now, here's the deal: if you miss a day, then immediately drop down to 4 minutes. If you miss two days in a row, drop back down to 3 minutes. Exercise is no longer a barrier because you've chosen to make it fun and easy.

Let's take a quick look at the exercises. Below you'll see the sets of exercises; core and total body.

TOTAL BODY	CORE
March in Place	Mountain Climber
Jumping Jacks	Planks
Air Squats	Inchworm
Squat Jacks	

EXERCISE LIBRARY:

Starting on the next page is a guide and photos for how to correctly do each exercise.

March in Place

In your walking shoes, start by walking in place at a pace that is comfortable for you. Swing your arms naturally by your side in pace with your marching. Lift knees up as much as is comfortable.

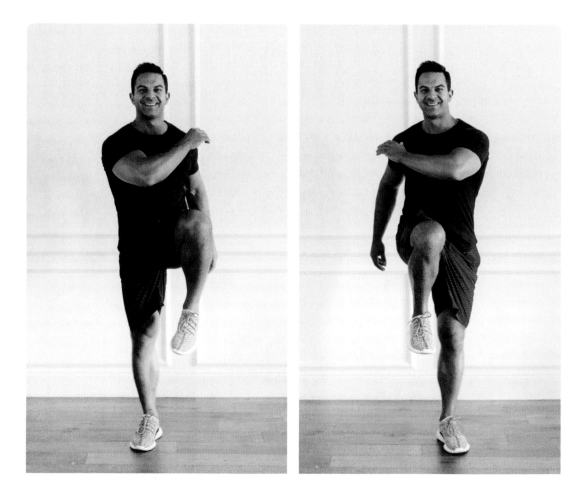

Jumping Jacks

Start with your feet together and your hands down by your side. Jump up into the air and land with your feet at shoulder-width apart and your hands touching above your head. Jump again back into starting position. Repeat.

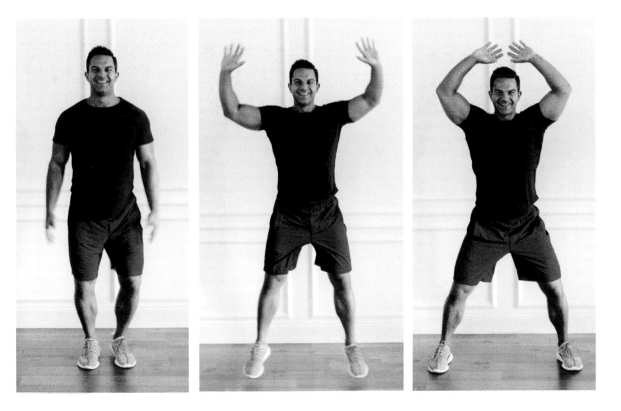

Air Squats

Start with your feet shoulder-width apart, toes slightly turned out, and your hands by your sides. Stretch your arms forward, bend at your knees, and push your butt back, as if you were sitting in a chair, until your thighs are parallel to the ground. Straighten your legs to come back up, while squeezing your butt, and return your arms back down to your sides. Repeat.

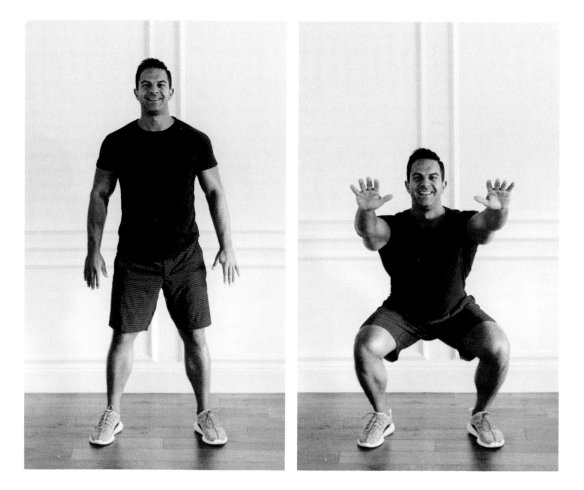

Squat Jack

Start with your feet together and your arms at your sides. Soft jump into a squat until your quads are about parallel to the ground. Keeping your weight on your heels, explode up through the balls of your feet and get a little bit of air underneath the feet. Softly land with your feet together, gently tapping the ground, and quickly repeat.

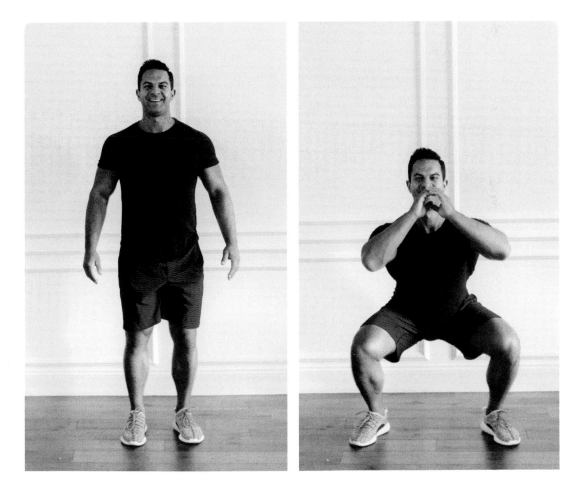

Mountain Climbers

Start down on the floor, with your arms straight off the ground, and your legs stretched out behind you in push-up position. Bring your right knee up to your right elbow, and then return your right foot back to starting position. Then bring your left knee to your left elbow and return your foot back to starting position. Repeat.

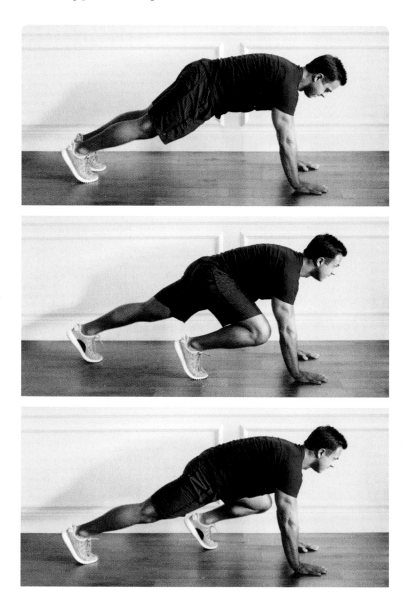

Planks

Start down on the floor, with your arms straight off the ground, and your legs stretched out behind you in push-up position. Bend at the elbows to lower yourself off your hands and onto your forearms, keeping your body straight from your shoulders to your ankles. Suck your belly button up towards your spine to engage your core, and hold that position for the set amount of time given.

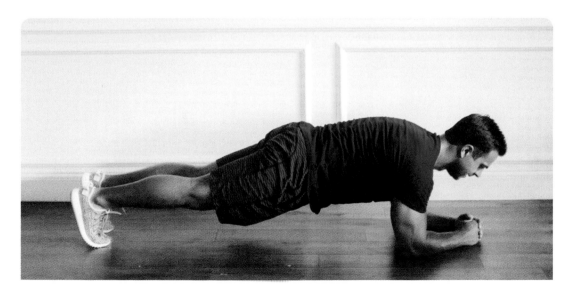

Inchworm

Start by standing with your feet shoulder-width apart and bend at the hips until your hands touch the ground. Walk your hands forward in front of your body until you are stretched out into push up position. Then, walk your hands back towards your feet until you are back at starting position.

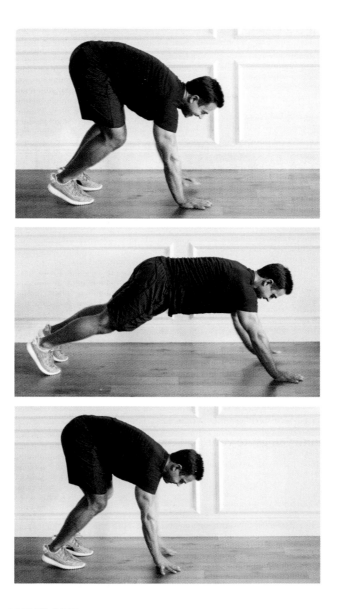

I have kept it very simple on purpose to remove barriers. The workouts are the same, 20 seconds on, 20 seconds off. You get to use any of the previous exercises to create your workout. Ideally, you would follow a total body exercise with a core exercise. It should look something like this.

Workout 1

MARCH IN PLACE—20 Seconds
REST—20 Seconds
MOUNTAIN CLIMBERS—20 Seconds
REST—20 seconds
GO RIGHT BACK INTO MARCHING IN PLACE—20 Seconds

And continue to repeat work/rest, work/rest for 3 minutes. As you progress, simply add work/rest intervals until you get to your goal time.

Workout 2

AIR SQUATS—20 Seconds
REST—20 Seconds
PLANK—20 Seconds
REST—20 seconds
GO RIGHT BACK INTO AIR SQUATS—20 Seconds

And continue to repeat work/rest, work/rest for 5 minutes. As you progress, simply add work/rest intervals until you get to your goal time.

If you need additional rest, all good, just take it. Just make a mental note of it and do your best to make progress every time you train.

That's all.

Now slam down a glass of water and get moving. And afterwards, you'll have energy you never knew you had that early in the morning. Just another bonus of firing up your metabolism first thing.

What's Next?

So what happens after you hit your first two exercise goals? Well, you move up (only if you choose). Level two is the exact same exercises, except this time you'll give me just five more minutes. That means you move up to ten total minutes a day, and if you choose to, you can break it up into two separate workouts.

You Are on Fire!

Alright you're cruising. You obviously want it really bad. You've nailed the above and you're ready for level three. Move up to 15 minutes and don't look back.

LEVEL 1: 3–5 minutes (1 session)
LEVEL 2: 10 minutes (1–2 sessions)
LEVEL 3: 15 minutes (1–3 sessions)

Keep Pushing!

After you've nailed 7 consecutive days at 15 minutes a day you can add another 15 minutes of any activity that you like. I encourage you to choose something you really like to do.

- Walk around the neighborhood
- Swim
- Hike an easy community trail
- Dance
- Deep clean your house (this really does work up a sweat)
- Rake leaves
- Build a snowman (Haha. I am from Wisconsin.)
- Play with your kids
- Kick a ball around at the park
- Play racquetball

Thirty minutes a day is a perfect amount of activity to keep your heart healthy, your stress low, and your body happy.

PS: I am really proud of you. Make sure to take some time to celebrate how far you've come. Your new habits are real, and you're in control. Be aware of how you're feeling in these moments, it's important, remember, it's your journey.

What If I Am Already Training?

You're already training, and you love to sweat. This section is for you, for those who already exercise on a regular basis. Here is where we can make some additional tweaks so you can get the most out of your carb cycle. Now, if you'd rather not worry about the details, then don't, because that's what these are. They WILL NOT make or break your efforts, only enhance them.

Structuring Your Training To Get the Most Out of Your Cycle

Like I said, these are the little details. If you like details, then here's how you can structure your workouts to get the most out of your nutrition. But first, let's give you some context as to why we do what we do and how your body uses fuel (food) for energy.

Fuel Sources During Exercise

Activity can be divided up into two categories:

INTENSE (PHOSOCREATINE AND ANAEROBIC/GLYCOLYTIC)

- Intense Weight Lifting
- High Intensity Interval or Cardio Training (ie: sprints)

This type of training is 90% or greater than your maximum output. This type of training isn't sustainable, but rather short, intense bursts. Think 0–120 seconds max.

MODERATE/LEISURE ACTIVITIES (AEROBIC)

- Cardio Training
- Day-to-Day Activities (running errands, cleaning, etc.)

This type of training is much lighter and sustainable for longer periods of time. Think 120 seconds and greater.

Your body utilizes fuel differently during these two types of training.

INTENSE TRAINING FUEL

When doing any form of very intense training, your body first utilizes glucose because it is the most immediate fuel source. Fat simply cannot be broken down fast enough to supply the necessary fuel to meet the demands of intense training.

HIGH CARBS MEANS HIGH ENERGY

Instead, your high-carb days should be reserved for your highest activity days, now that means something different to everyone based on their current level of fitness. So, with that in mind, listen to your body and schedule you most intense training days (if you train), or your highest activity days (if you don't train) around your high carb meals/days. I also always use the medium- and high-carb days to get my critical thinking tasks done, too. Your brain uses up more glycogen than any other part of your body, so don't wait for your low- and no-carb days to get projects done that require lots of brain juice.

Doing intense training on medium-carb days is fine, you should still have sufficient fuel to get through the workout. And on medium-carb days, you can time your carbs by consuming them just before (1hr) and after your workout (within 1hr).

HIGH-CARB DAYS (WITH REWARD MEAL)

Here's what I do: I set up my workouts to fall right before the reward meal on a high-carb day, and boy do I earn it. This way my muscles are primed for the extra carbohydrates. Or, if it's a strength day, the day after I went ham (pun intended!). You will be surprised at how much stronger your lifts are post-reward meal day.

Post-workout your body will immediately start replenishing muscle glycogen reserves and help kick-start the rebuilding process. Plus, after a hard session, you'll notice that your reward meal tastes much better, at least I do! There's something about earning it that makes it taste even more delicious.

Save your most intense training/activity days for high-carb days. Carb-up prior to your workout, too. Include a good amount of slow carbohydrates (aka sweet potatoes) about an hour before your workout and you will feel the difference in your training capacity, guaranteed! For example, legs are my most intense day, so I reserve my high-carb reward day for leg day.

MEDIUM-CARB DAYS

Feel out your medium carb days. There have been times where I have trained legs on my medium-carb days, too. The workouts are usually not as intense, but still good enough. The reality is, sometimes you'll have to make adjustments. Remember, it's not black and white.

Those of you doing HIIT (high-intensity interval training), like my best selling HIIT MAX™ program (morellifit.com/hiit-max), should be able to push through a 15-20-minute session, no problem.

LOW-CARB DAYS

Note that with the Activate Hot and Accelerated Inferno Cycles, you'll likely need to do one or two workouts per week on a low-carb day. Do your best, nothing more, and nothing less, and you will find great success with or without these little details.

Remember, you have "Four Types of Carb Days," and you get to enjoy a portion of carbs, even on low-carb days. You can always prioritize your carbohydrates right before and after your workouts. This means you can move your meals around to fit your training schedule. This will allow you to work at your highest capacity during your workouts.

A NO-NO ON NO-CARB DAYS

Attempting to do intense training, such as heavy weight lifting or high-intensity intervals, on your no-carb day will more often than not be a serious struggle. I usually rest or do some light aerobic work on my no-carb days, and I suggest the same for you.

Example Training/Cycle Schedule

Here is just one of many examples on how you might structure your training around your carbs. Remember, "intense" means something different to everyone. Listen to your body and set up your highest activity days around your highest carb days.

HIGH-CARB DAY: Most Intense Training Day
MEDIUM-CARB DAY: Moderate Intense Training Day
LOW-CARB DAY: Lighter Intense Training
NO-CARB DAY: Rest/Recovery Day

Now, let's get real to talk about pre/post-workout nutrition and supplementation. In the next chapter, we'll discuss how you can time your nutrition and supplementation to get the biggest bang for your buck. Don't worry, if you're not there yet it's all good. Again, these are the finer details and something to work towards on your journey.

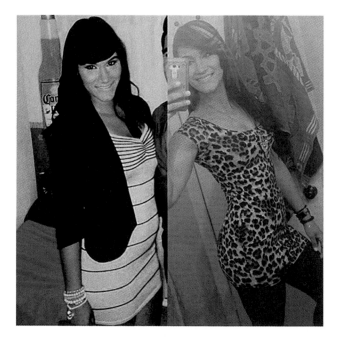

 דניאלה (@srtadanielle)

I wont go back progress #littlebylittle #workout #fit #healthy #gym #fitness #nevergiveup #planetfitness #fitcouple #sweetpotatodiet #nutritionplan #jimstoppani #bodybuilder #bodybuilding #motivation

3:23pm 06/06/2016 6 ♥ 65

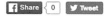

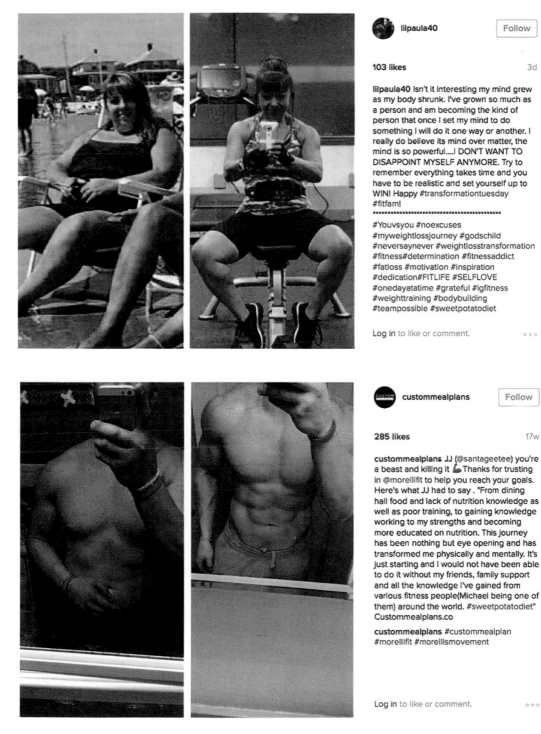

lilpaula40 Follow

103 likes 3d

lilpaula40 Isn't it interesting my mind grew as my body shrunk. I've grown so much as a person and am becoming the kind of person that once I set my mind to do something I will do it one way or another. I really do believe its mind over matter, the mind is so powerful....I DON'T WANT TO DISAPPOINT MYSELF ANYMORE. Try to remember everything takes time and you have to be realistic and set yourself up to WIN! Happy #transformationtuesday #fitfam!
••
#Youvsyou #noexcuses #myweightlossjourney #godschild #neversaynever #weightlosstransformation #fitness#determination #fitnessaddict #fatloss #motivation #inspiration #dedication#FITLIFE #SELFLOVE #onedayatatime #grateful #igfitness #weighttraining #bodybuilding #teampossible #sweetpotatodiet

Log in to like or comment. ○○○

custommealplans Follow

285 likes 17w

custommealplans JJ (@santageetee) you're a beast and killing it 💪Thanks for trusting in @morellifit to help you reach your goals. Here's what JJ had to say . "From dining hall food and lack of nutrition knowledge as well as poor training, to gaining knowledge working to my strengths and becoming more educated on nutrition. This journey has been nothing but eye opening and has transformed me physically and mentally. It's just starting and I would not have been able to do it without my friends, family support and all the knowledge I've gained from various fitness people(Michael being one of them) around the world. #sweetpotatodiet" Custommealplans.co

custommealplans #custommealplan #morellifit #morellismovement

Log in to like or comment. ○○○

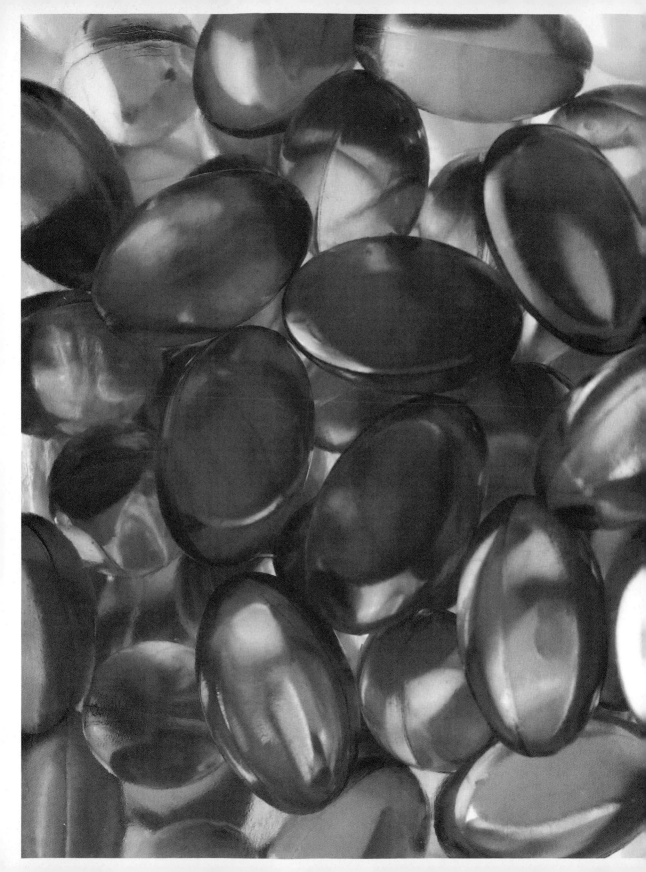

CHAPTER 17

Timing Your Nutrition and Supplementation

There's one last thing to cover—keep in mind, this wasn't something I did right out of the gate. While I do feel it's important, it's not the most important. What's most important is that you take action and build consistency with your daily food intake. When you're ready, the benefits of proper timing and supplementation ensure the next level of success.

There Are Two Critical Times

Before and after your workout are the two most critical times for fueling your body. One gives your body the fuel to work out, and the other is the fuel to repair and build right after a workout.

When you can, I suggest eating and/or supplementing an hour or so prior to training and within an hour post-workout. The idea behind nutrient timing is to manipulate the hormones affected by food as well as the hormones affected by training.

What Does This Mean?

Timing is a way to take your fitness success to the next level. How your body utilizes a baked potato is different based on whether it is eaten at night for dinner or immediately after your training.

Why Does This Happen?

Post-workout, your glycogen stores are depleted and your body's insulin sensitivity is extremely high, which means your body is ready to shuttle the fuel you consume directly into the muscles. This leads to fast recovery and better nutrient uptake for protein.

Pre-Workout Nutrition Timing

The general rule of thumb for pre-workout nutrition is to eat some complex carbohydrates along with some lean protein. This is something you will have to feel out. Some people cannot eat a meal an hour before training, so this is where a shake might work best.

If you eat your pre-workout meal at least two hours prior to your workout session, then you can also add some healthy fats such as avocado, nuts, or nut butters. This healthy fat will also help to slow the digestion process, helping you avoid a blood sugar crash partway through your workout session.

A lot of it is oftentimes trial and error, because everybody is different and responds to food and supplementation differently. Try a few different things over the course of a couple weeks and be aware of how you feel. Proceed with what makes you feel best.

Post-Workout Nutrition Timing

Refueling after a workout session is critical.

What you do in that session should dictate how you refuel. With the goal of fat loss, we need to be careful not to overdo the post-workout carbs. Follow your cycle.

Your post-workout refuel should be one of your meals for the day. Make sure you eat it as soon as you can post-workout. Muscle protein synthesis is at its peak just after a workout and starts to diminish every hour, so choosing to eat as soon as you can gives you the most bang for your workout. You don't need to run any red lights to get home, do your best and get your meal in as soon as you can.

What If I Train Late at Night?

This is one question I get every day on social media. Many people think that if they train late they should skip the carbs—no! 1000% absolutely not. You must always eat carbs post-workout, it's the law. Does that mean you need some carbs after going on a walk around the block, no. But if you train with any sort of intensity, especially HIIT or weight training, then you get some carbs in. Sweet potatoes are the best late at night, especially if your goal is fat loss, as they won't spike your blood sugar before bed.

The Key Supplements

It's almost impossible to get all of the nutrients we need out of the food we consume. There's a lot of supplements I don't agree with, and so my list is short and sweet. I am not an advocate of meal replacements or fat burners and I do not think you have any business supplementing if you haven't first taken a look at and done your best with your diet and training. There's no supplementation in the world that's going to outwork a shit diet, period. It will always be whole foods from as close to nature as possible. Now, with that in mind, here are some of the supplements I strongly advise in order to get the most out of your training and nutrition. They are not in any order of importance, and some I offer and some I don't.

1. PROTEIN

Getting enough protein is important. Most people have a hard time consuming enough protein for their needs, I certainly do. I do not ever replace whole food meals, I only use protein to supplement or when I am on-the-go and something is better than nothing. If you're like me and you do need supplements, please make sure that you choose wisely. I would never, ever take anything that wasn't 100% grass-fed and flash pasteurized. It's cleaner and more bioavailable, which means your body will absorb and utilize it far more than inferior types of protein powders. I spent two years formulating ours, it has only 5 total ingredients and is sourced from grass-fed cows out of New Zealand. You can learn more about it here—www.morellifit .com/whey-protein

2. FISH OR KRILL OIL

Fish oil is another important supplement that I believe everyone should take regularly no matter what. It's great for cognitive health, joint health, and hair and skin regeneration. It also fights inflammation. I strongly advise a krill oil, it's far better quality and offers some very worthwhile added benefits. With this in mind, it's important to get Omega-3 and 6s in your diet through whole food. You'll never get enough, so a supplement here is necessary. You can learn more about our krill oil at www.morellifit.com/krill-oil.

3. PROBIOTICS

A good probiotic is a must, period. Probiotics are live bacteria and yeasts that are good for your health, especially your digestive system. They are often called "good" or "helpful" bacteria because they help keep your gut healthy. You can get live probiotics from a number of foods and drink and I strongly encourage that you do. Things such as; kefir, dark chocolate, kombucha, sauerkraut, and kimchi contain probiotics. Your body naturally has bacteria in it, both good and bad, and the good bacteria help to keep your gut healthy. This is what a probiotic is. Probiotics are live microorganisms that work to keep your gut happy and healthy.

A good probiotic also supports a healthy immune system. When choosing a good probiotic, you need to make sure that it has multiple strains of bacteria and that they are diverse, with some of the most important being *lactobacillus* and *bifidobacterium* (or L and B) strains. These strains support your large and small intestines. Your probiotic supplement should also clearly state how many CFUs (colony forming units) are in the bottle, and it should be clearly labeled as a guarantee, so you know the CFU count up until the expiration date. Potency can decrease as time goes on. We don't offer a probiotic just yet, the one I currently take is Dr. Ohhira's Probiotics Professional Formula.

4. BCAAs, AKA BRANCH CHAIN AMINO ACIDS

What can I say? I am a fan of BCAAs. If you follow me on any of the social media platforms, you'll see me sipping them all day, and for a number of reasons. BCAAs are comprised of leucine, isoleucine, and valine and are chained together to form peptides. These peptides are responsible for a number of things, including muscle preservation and muscle protein synthesis. They are great for recovery, and when you sip on them during your training, they will extend the rate of perceived exertion. In simple terms this means you don't get tired as fast and can oftentimes push through the most intense workouts. They are also exceptionally good to drink throughout your low- and no-carb day as they have been shown to ward off hunger, and since you're in a deficit or catabolic state on these days, they work to preserve your lean muscle tissue which is a must. With that in mind, drink something really clean, something without artificial flavors, dyes, colors, or added fillers, and preferably without sucrose or other harmful sugars. I worked really hard to finally launch a formula that tastes great (like an orange dreamsicle) and that was sucralose free without any of the crap I just mentioned. You can learn more about our brand here: www.morellifit.com/bcaas

5. PRE-WORKOUT

Pre-workouts are just not my thing, way too many ingredients and garbage in them for my liking. I have not seen one clean enough to put into my body, so for the last three years or so I just take a double shot of espresso or drink an 8 oz glass of black coffee. Most people don't know that coffee will give you all the kick you need to push through the most intense training, and everyone that has taken my word for it always says the same thing. "Wow, Michael!" Coffee contains caffeine as you know, and caffeine is actually the number one most underutilized fat burner on the market in its natural form. It's all you need. Something you should know, is coffee is the most heavily-sprayed crop on the planet, so always go local, and always go organic. I don't drink it otherwise. I have had a passion for coffee for a very long time, so much so that I partnered with a farm in Costa Rica, San Rafael, and made my own brand (*haha* I know, I know). It's the best, like all of my stuff it's organic, fair trade, and has unbelievable taste. It's a dark roast that you can drink black all day long, but don't. I suggest only 1–2 cups per day. I consume a cup in the morning and a cup before my workout, depending on whether or not I need a boost. You can learn more here (if you choose)—www.morelliscoffee.com

Hey, can you blame me? I found all of the holes in the supplement industry and created better. I was sick and tired of putting crap in my body, and now I don't have to do that anymore. Do your research and decide what's best for you, always.

Energy-Boosting Solutions

I know that on low-carb and no-carb days, I need to reach for a little extra energy. On these days, I sip on Morellifit Nutrition BCAAs. Consider sipping on some BCAAs (branched chain amino acids) during your workout on all training days. They will give you a little more energy to get through your workout on low-carb days and help protect against lean muscle mass loss.

On lower-carb days, a shot of espresso can give an additional energy boost. This is good

30 minutes prior to a workout. And, if you're really struggling, a small banana may be required instead. Just keep in mind that the banana will add carbs, so your day will wind up not being quite as low on carbs as intended. But I think if eating a small banana means doing the workout versus skipping it, then it's better to eat it and go work out.

USING PROTEIN SUPPLEMENTS

If you are considering supplementing with protein, look for something that's naturally sweetened (or unsweetened) with as few ingredients as possible. Morellifit Nutrition is my supplement brand and is a solid choice when it comes to amino acids. Look for:

- Grass-fed whey protein
- Pure whey protein isolate
- For vegetarians, rice or pea protein (stay away from soy and corn)

WORDS OF CAUTION: We always suggest getting your protein sources from whole foods first, but we know that sometimes when you are on the run, it is more convenient to have something that you can just take and drink. Remember, if you have a protein shake as a meal, you will need to include the portions of carbs (if any) for the day. This is where good fruits come in handy. The same goes for fats in that meal—peanut butter or flax seed would be great additions to the smoothie. Don't leave out any of the parts of your meal just because you are consuming it differently.

And that's precisely how you can dial in pre- and post-workout nutrition while keeping your carb cycle intact.

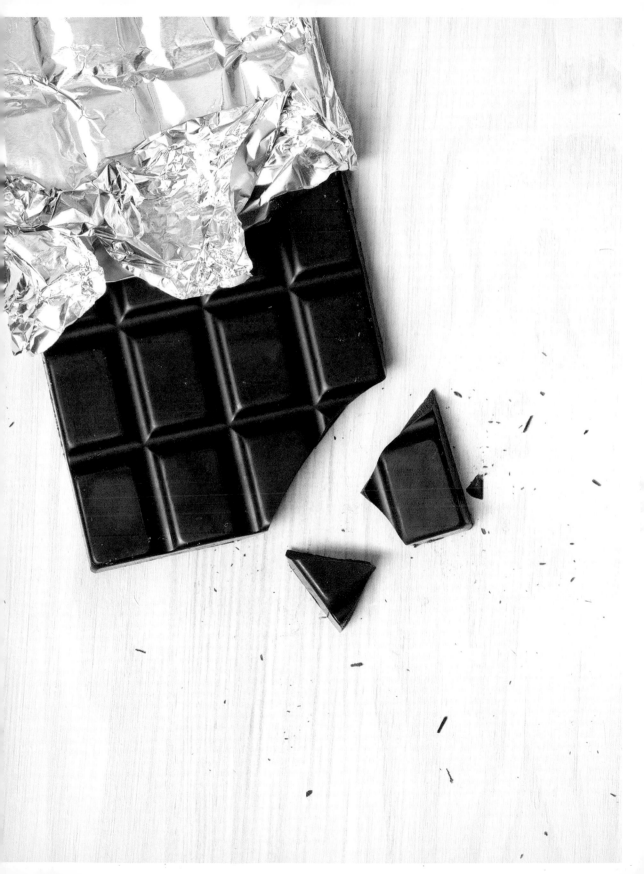

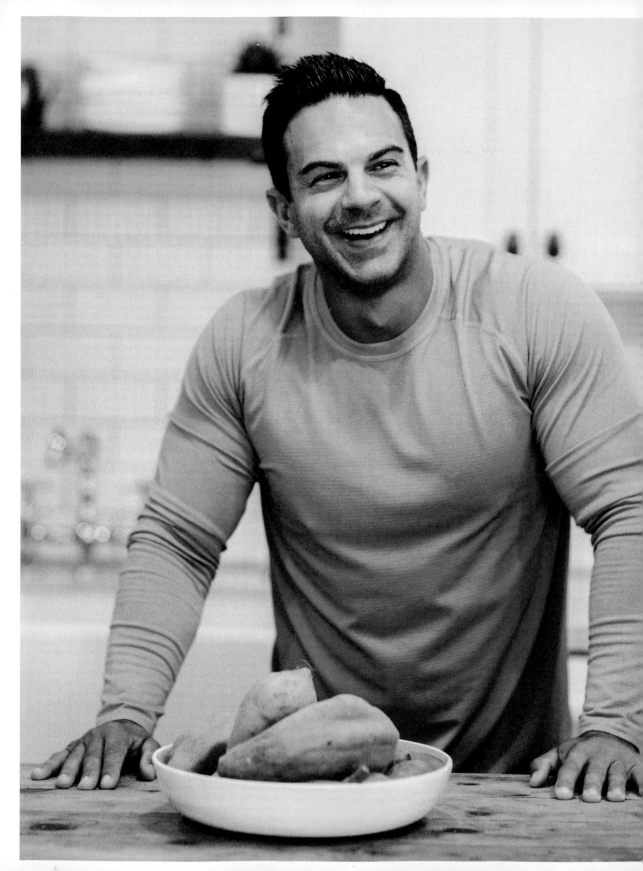

CHAPTER 18:

Taking Control

Making It Happen

The Sweet Potato Diet was carefully designed over a number of years to deliver noticeable, rapid, and lasting fat loss...if you take action. You cannot win without action. Many times easier said than done for a number of reasons; limiting beliefs, self-worth, fear of failure, and emotional attachment to food are the first that come to mind. I know how you feel, I have been on anti-depressants, I have failed with numerous diets, and I have felt many times over that I am just not worthy of a phenomenal physique. Maybe you're like I was, where you've tried countless times in the past without success and now feel as though every diet is the same and none of them work. I can assure you that's not the case with the Sweet Potato Diet. It has worked, and continues to work for thousands of people all over the world. It will work if you use it, and action is the key ingredient—period.

Giving up, Getting Sick, and Dying

Take action now if you haven't already. Free yourself from the nonstop futile dieting that most people painfully endure year after year until they give up, get sick, or experience a premature death. I am sorry if that's too blunt, but it's the truth. We oftentimes only place value on our health once we begin to lose it. Is that what it's going to take? You think this is hard now, how hard do you think it would be if, God forbid, you had diabetes or heart disease? And if you're reading this and that's you right now, it could always be worse. I just met a guy by the name of Pat (@possiblepat on Instagram). He was pre-diabetic and 605 pounds two years ago. I found out after following much of my advice (eating lots of sweet potatoes) and tons of his own hard work, he lost 340 pounds—insane right?! So, what's different about him? He's got kids, a sixty-hour-a-week job, and he still did it. He didn't even have the step-by-step blueprint that you're holding in your hand.

So, what's it gonna be? Are you going to end up just another statistic? Or are you going to fucking fight with me, with us?! The entire morellifit community is here to support you. I am surely not going to give up on you! Not now, not ever!

Pain Today Equals Strength Tomorrow!

It's going to be hard, you will get frustrated, and you will think about giving up. Remember, your greatest pains become your biggest strengths, and the more adversity you overcome, the more resilient you become. What you're made of today isn't what you'll be made of tomorrow, and through your experiences come purpose, passion, fulfillment and often lead to a cause greater than you.

I am a perfect example of that, and I know hundreds, if not thousands of others who have used some pain in their life to reach others in need. Who will you reach? Who will you lead? What example are you to those closest to you? And lastly, what do you want people to say at your funeral? Now you're thinking…good. That was my intention. You were destined for greatness, we all were, the sad part is that most of us die without ever figuring out what that is. Your new journey is the gateway, and it's going to open some incredible doors for you.

All those painful struggles, trials, and errors I had over the years led to this book. What will your journey lead you to accomplish? You don't need to answer that question now. We have just manifested it, it will come in time and through experiences.

I am grateful you've given me the opportunity to join you on your journey through my book. All you need to do now is meet me halfway and follow it, as it's laid out, and if you need me drop me a line on your favorite social media platform. I will always do my best to get back to you. And if I miss it, continue reaching out until I see it—please. I am here for you. I am all in.

The Support You Need, Right Here

Throw out the excuses. And if you haven't fully committed: NOW IS THE TIME!

Give yourself 100% for the next thirty days only, and if at the end of the first thirty you don't feel like it's worth it to continue, quit.

Deal?

Yes, I am giving you permission to quit after thirty days if you don't feel like it's worth it to continue, under one condition, you give me 100% for the entire time.

If you don't already know me online, you'll find that I give away tons of valuable, free information on my blog and social media channels. There is a wealth of information on my channels as well as one huge family that loves unconditionally through both success and setback.

You can sign up to get my free newsletter, where I dish out cutting-edge information and share all of my new heath hacks. Get involved, trust me. The extra support, motivation, and accountability will undoubtedly get you to the next level. I am so excited for you!

Please join us here—www.morellifit.com.

To Your Health,
Michael Morelli Jr.

Appendix: Food Log / Meal Planner

	MONDAY	TUESDAY	WEDNESD
BREAKFAST			
MORNING SNACK			
LUNCH			
AFTERNOON SNACK			
DINNER			
NIGHTTIME SNACK			
WATER	○○○○○ ○○○○○ ○○○○○	○○○○○ ○○○○○ ○○○○○	○○○○○ ○○○○○ ○○○○○

THURSDAY	FRIDAY	SATURDAY	SUNDAY
○○○○○ ○○○○○ ○○○○○	○○○○○ ○○○○○ ○○○○○	○○○○○ ○○○○○ ○○○○○	○○○○○ ○○○○○ ○○○○○

References

Introduction

What's New and Beneficial about Sweet Potatoes. Retrieved December 30, 2015, from http://www.whfoods.org/genpage.php?tname=foodspice&dbid=64.

Powell, C. (2012). *Choose to lose: The 7-day carb cycle solution.* New York: Hyperion.

Pharmaceutical Industry. (2015). Retrieved December 30, 2015, from http://www.who.int/trade/glossary/story073/en/.

Keesler, C. (2011, April 15). Sweet Potato (Ipomoea batatas). Retrieved January 11, 2016, from http://bioweb.uwlax.edu/bio203/2011/keesler_cole/.

Ugent, D., & Peterson, L. W. (1988). Archaeological remains of potato and sweet potato in Peru. *CIP Circular.*

Hirst, K. Why is the American Sweet Potato History Connected to Polynesia? Retrieved December 8, 2015, from http://archaeology.about.com/od/domestications/qt/sweet_potato.htm.

O'Brien, P. J. (1972). The Sweet Potato: Its Origin and Dispersal. *American Anthropologist,* 74(3), 342–365.

Gerard, J., & Rogers, W. (1597). *The herball, or, Generall historie of plantes.* Imprinted at London: By Iohn Norton.

A Sweet Potato History. (2011). Retrieved December 8, 2015, from http://blogs.loc.gov/inside_adams/2010/11/a-sweet-potato-history.

Carver, G. (1936). *How the farmer can save his sweet potatoes: And ways of preparing them for the table* (4th ed.). Tuskegee, Ala.: Tuskegee Institute Press.

Tudor, A. (2012). *Sweet potato power: Smart carbs, paleo and personalized.* Las Vegas, Nev.: Victory Belt Pub.

McGreger, A. (2014). *Sweet potatoes.* The University of North Carolina Press.

Beat the Odds

Ogden, C., Carroll, M., Kit, B., & Flegal, K. (2014). Prevalence of Childhood and Adult Obesity in the United States, 2011–2012. *Survey of Anesthesiology,* 206-206.

How Our Diet Went Wrong

Blasco, R., Rosell, J., Cuartero, F., Peris, J. F., Gopher, A., & Barkai, R. (2014). Correction: Using Bones to Shape Stones: MIS 9 Bone Retouchers at Both Edges of the Mediterranean Sea. *PloS one,* 9(1).

Richards, M. P. (2002). A brief review of the archaeological evidence for Palaeolithic and Neolithic subsistence. *European Journal of Clinical Nutrition,* 56(12), 16-p.

Francis, R. (2007). Anti-Cancer Diet. Retrieved from http://beyondhealth.com/media/wysiwyg/kadro/articles/Anti-cancerDiet.pdf.

World Health Organization. (Urban population growth. Retrieved December 7, 2015, from http://www.who.int/gho/urban_health/situation_trends/urban_population_growth_text/en/.

Ervin, R. B., & Ogden, C. L. (2013). Consumption of added sugars among US adults, 2005-2010. NCHS *data brief,* (122), 1-8.

Decker, E. A., & Park, Y. (2010). Healthier meat products as functional foods. *Meat Science,* 86(1), 49-55.

MacDonald, G. (2010). Identification of Health and Nutritional Benefits of New Zealand Aquaculture Seafood's. *Report to Aquaculture New Zealand.*

The University of Michigan Health System. (2009). Retrieved December 31, 2015, from http://www.med.umich.edu/umim/food-pyramid/eggs.html.

Hoernle, N. (2015). You Are What You Eat. Retrieved December 31, 2015, from http://www.granitemedical.com/health_education/ounce_prevention/you-are-what-you-eat.cfm.

Avoid the Most Damaging Weight Loss Myths Most People Believe

Brand-Miller, J. (2013, April 2). Good Carbs, Bad Carbs. Retrieved December 31, 2015, from http://www.obesityaustralia.org/general-public-fact-sheets/good-carbs-bad-carbs.

Bachman, J. L., Phelan, S., Wing, R. R., & Raynor, H. A. (2011). Eating frequency is higher in weight loss maintainers and normal-weight individuals than in overweight individuals. *Journal of the American Dietetic Association,* 111(11), 1730-1734.

National Institute of Allergy and Infectious Diseases. (2014). Weight-loss and Nutrition Myths (NIH Publication No. 04–4561). Retrieved from http://www.niddk.nih.gov/health-information/health-topics/weight-control/myths/Documents/Myths.pdf

Vreeman, R. C., & Carroll, A. E. (2008). Festive medical myths. *BMJ, 337,* a2769.

Andrews, R. (2012). All About Carb Cycling. Retrieved from http://www.precisionnutrition.com/all-about-carb-cycling.

Healthy Snacking. (2014). Retrieved January 12, 2016, from http://www.heart.org/HEARTORG/Getting-Healthy/NutritionCenter/HealthyCooking/Healthy-Snacking_UCM_301489_Article.jsp#.VpWCrpMrL-Y.

Vella, C. A., & Kravitz, L. (2004). Exercise after-burn: A research update. *IDEA Fitness Journal, 1*(5), 42-47.

Mind Mastery for Lasting Weight Loss

Cheren, M., Foushi, M., Gudmundsdotter, E., Hillock, C., Lerner, M., Prager, M., . . . Werdell, P. (2009). Food Addiction Institute. Retrieved December 7, 2015, from http://foodaddictioninstitute.org/scientific-research/physical-craving-and-food-addiction-a-scientific-review.

Blackman, M. (2008). *Mind your diet: The psychology behind sticking to any diet.* Philadelphia, PA: Xlibris.

Weir, K., & Carter, W. J. (2011). The exercise effect. *Monitor on Psychology/APA, 42,* 48.

The Surprising Role Integrity Plays in Your Battle Against Fat

"Visualization" Brings Home the Gold for Olympian Gymnast Gabby Douglas. (2002, August 7). Retrieved December 8, 2015, from http://www.prweb.com/releases/2012/8/prweb9766570.htm.

Lustig, R. (2012, February 21). The Most Unhappy of Pleasures: This Is Your Brain on Sugar. Retrieved December 31, 2015, from http://www.theatlantic.com/health/archive/2012/02/the-most-unhappy-of-pleasures-this-is-your-brain-on-sugar/253341/.

Courage, K. (2014, March 19). Why Is Dark Chocolate Good for You? Thank Your Microbes. Retrieved December 31, 2015, from http://www.scientificamerican.com/article/why-is-dark-chocolate-good-for-you-thank-your-microbes/.

SMART and Easy Ways That Help You Knock Out Fat

Matthews, G. (2013). Goals Research Summary. Retrieved December 31, 2015, from http://www.dominican.edu/academics/ahss/undergraduate-programs/psych/faculty/assets-gail-matthews/researchsummary2.pdf.

Victory Is Yours…If You Prepare for It

Bray, G., Nielsen, S., & Popkin, B. (2004). Consumption of high-fructose corn syrup in beverages may play a role in the epidemic of obesity. *The American Journal of Clinical Nutrition, 79*(4), 537-543.

Malik, V. S., Popkin, B. M., Bray, G. A., Després, J. P., Willett, W. C., & Hu, F. B. (2010). Sugar-sweetened beverages and risk of metabolic syndrome and type 2 diabetes A meta-analysis. *Diabetes Care, 33*(11), 2477-2483.

Lennerz, B., Alsop, D., Holsen, L., Stern, E., Rojas, R., Ebbeling, C., . . . Ludwig, D. (2013). Effects of dietary glycemic index on brain regions related to reward and craving in men. *American Journal of Clinical Nutrition,* 641-647.

Waring, B. (2014, April 11). Visualizing Future May Help Weight Loss, Epstein Says - The NIH Record - April 11, 2014. Retrieved December 8, 2015, from https://nihrecord.nih.gov/newsletters/2014/04_11_2014/story1.htm.

Christakis, N. A., & Fowler, J. H. (2007). The spread of obesity in a large social network over 32 years. *New England journal of medicine, 357*(4), 370-379.

Poirier, P., Giles, T., Bray, G., Hong, Y., Stern, J., Pi-Sunyer, X., & Eckel, R. (2006). Obesity and Cardiovascular Disease: Pathophysiology, Evaluation, and Effect of Weight Loss: An Update of the 1997 American Heart Association Scientific Statement on Obesity and Heart Disease From the Obesity Committee of the Council on Nutrition, Physical. *Circulation,* 898-918.

Switch It Up: Why Variety Is Important

Arimond, M., & Ruel, M. T. (2004). Dietary diversity is associated with child nutritional status: evidence from 11 demographic and health surveys. *The Journal of Nutrition, 134*(10), 2579-2585.

National Institute of Allergy and Infectious Diseases. (2012). Food Allergy: An Overview (NIH Publication No. 12-5518). Retrieved from https://www.niaid.nih.gov/topics/foodAllergy/Documents/foodallergy.pdf.

How to Hydrate for Fat Loss

Juan, W., & Basiotis, P. P. (2004). More than one in three older Americans may not drink enough water. *Family Economics and Nutrition Review, 16*(1), 49.

Barron, J. (2014, August 4). Digestive Enzymes for a Modern Diet. Retrieved January 5, 2016, from http://jonbarron.org/digestive-health/digestive-enzymes-healthy-diet#.VowmlZMrJsN.

Davy, B. M., Dennis, E. A., Dengo, A. L., Wilson, K. L., & Davy, K. P. (2008). Water Consumption Reduces Energy Intake at a Breakfast Meal in Obese Older Adults. *Journal of the American Dietetic Association, 108*(7), 1236–1239. http://doi.org/10.1016/j.jada.2008.04.013

Spriet, L., & Graham, T. Caffeine and Exercise Performance. *American College of Sports Medicine.* Retrieved December 8, 2015, from http://www.acsm.org/docs/current-comments/caffeineandexercise.pdf.

Mitchell, T. (2006). Theanine: Natural support for sleep, mood, and weight. *Life Extension Magazine.*

Janson, M. (2008). HEALTHY LIVING. *Dr. Michael Janson's Healthy Living,* 8(4), 1-4. Retrieved from http://www.drjanson.com/djhl-pdf/2006/DJHL-2006-04.pdf

Lieber, C. S., & Schmid, R. (1961). The Effect of Ethanol on Fatty Acid METABOLISM; STIMULATION OF HEPATIC FATTY ACID SYNTHESIS *IN VITRO. Journal of Clinical Investigation,* 40(2), 394–399.

Emanuele, M. A., & Emanuele, N. (2001). Alcohol and the male reproductive system. *Alcohol Research and Health,* 25(4), 282-287.

Scanlan, M. F., Roebuck, T., Little, P. J., & Naughton, M. T. (2000). Effect of moderate alcohol upon obstructive sleep apnoea. *European Respiratory Journal,* 16(5), 909-913.

Emanuele, N., & Emanuele, M. A. (1996). The endocrine system: alcohol alters critical hormonal balance. *Alcohol Health and Research World,* 21(1), 53-64.

Nilsson, M., Stenberg, M., Frid, A. H., Holst, J. J., & Björck, I. M. (2004). Glycemia and insulinemia in healthy subjects after lactose-equivalent meals of milk and other food proteins: the role of plasma amino acids and incretins. *The American Journal of Clinical Nutrition,* 80(5), 1246-1253.

Ludwig, D. S., & Willett, W. C. (2013). Three daily servings of reduced-fat milk: an evidence-based recommendation, *JAMA Pediatrics,* 167(9), 788-789.

Berkey, C. S., Rockett, H. R., Willett, W. C., & Colditz, G. A. (2005). Milk, dairy fat, dietary calcium, and weight gain: a longitudinal study of adolescents. *Archives of Pediatrics & Adolescent Medicine,* 159(6), 543-550.

The Secret Weapon for Successful Weight Loss (It's Not What You Think)

National Heart, Lung, and Blood Institute. Portion Distortion II Interactive Quiz. Retrieved from http://www.nhlbi.nih.gov/health/educational/wecan/portion/documents/PD2.pdf.

Proteins: The Most Essential Nutrient

Nesheim, M., & Nestle, M. (2012, September 20). Is a Calorie a Calorie? Retrieved December 31, 2015, from http://www.pbs.org/wgbh/nova/body/is-a-calorie-a-calorie.html.

What's so super about superfoods? (2013, November 1). Retrieved December 8, 2015, from http://www.heart.org/HEARTORG/GettingHealthy/NutritionCenter/HealthyDietGoals/Whats-so-super-about-superfoods_UCM_457937_Article.jsp#.VmcSUOODGko.

Castaneda, C., Charnley, J. M., Evans, W. J., & Crim, M. C. (1995). Elderly women accommodate to a low-protein diet with losses of body cell mass, muscle function, and immune response. *The American Journal of Clinical Nutrition, 62*(1), 30-39.

Paddon-Jones, D., Westman, E., Mattes, R., Wolfe, R., Astrup, A., & Westerterp-Plantenga, M. (2008). Protein, weight management, and satiety. *American Journal of Clinical Nutrition, 87*(5), 1558S-1561S.

Bilsborough, S., & Mann, N. (2006). A review of issues of dietary protein intake in humans. *International Journal of Sport Nutrition and Exercise Metabolism, 16*(2), 129.

Dietary Reference Intakes for Energy, Carbohydrate, Fiber, Fat, Fatty Acids, Cholesterol, Protein, and Amino Acids. (2005). Washington, DC: National Academies Press.

Carbs: Using Them Wisely

Carbohydrates: Complex Carbs vs Simple Carbs. (2015, July 9). Retrieved January 4, 2016, from http://www.pcrm.org/health/diets/recipes/complex-carbohydrates-vs-simple-carbohydrates.

Carbohydrates and Blood Sugar. Retrieved January 4, 2016, from http://www.hsph.harvard.edu/nutrition source/carbohydrates/carbohydrates-and-blood-sugar/.

Background on Carbohydrates & Sugars. Retrieved January 4, 2016, from http://www.foodinsight.org/Background_on_Carbohydrates_Sugars.

The science behind the sweetness in our diets. (2014). *Bulletin of the World Health Organization Bull. World Health Organization,* 780-781.

Fats: More Essential Than You Think

Ricciotti, E, FitzGerald, G.A. Prostaglandins and Inflammation. *Arteriosclerosis, Thrombosis, and Vascular Biology.* 2011;31(5):986-1000. doi:10.1161/ATVBAHA.110.207449.

Bhasin, S., Storer, T. W., Berman, N., Callegari, C., Clevenger, B., Phillips, J. ... & Casaburi, R. (1996). The effects of supraphysiologic doses of testosterone on muscle size and strength in normal men. *New England Journal of Medicine, 335*(1), 1-7.

Nutrition Basics. Retrieved January 5, 2016, from http://mynutrition.wsu.edu/nutrition-basics/.

Bellows, L., & Moore, R. (2012, November 1). Fat-Soluble Vitamins: A, D, E, and K – 9.315. Retrieved January 5, 2016, from http://extension.colostate.edu/topic-areas/nutrition-food-safety-health/fat-soluble-vitamins-a-d-e-and-k-9-315/.

Types of Fat. Retrieved December 8, 2015, from http://www.hsph.harvard.edu/nutritionsource/types-of-fat/.

Pham-Huy LA, He H, Pham-Huy C. Free Radicals, Antioxidants in Disease and Health. *International Journal of Biomedical Science* : IJBS. 2008;4(2):89-96.

Dean, W., & English, J. (2013, April 22). Medium Chain Triglycerides (MCTs): Beneficial Effects on Energy, Atherosclerosis and Aging. Retrieved January 5, 2016, from http://nutritionreview.org/2013/04/medium-chain-triglycerides-mcts/.

Fat composition of beef & sheepmeat: Opportunities for manipulation. (2008). *Meat Technology Update,* 1-4. Retrieved January 5, 2016, from http://www.meatupdate.csiro.au/data/MEAT_TECHNOLOGY_UPDATE_08-2.pdf.

Comparison of muscle fatty acid profiles and cholesterol concentrations of bison, beef, cattle, elk, and chicken. (2002). *Journal of Animal Science,* 80, 1202-1211.

Duda, M., O'shea, K., Tintinu, A., Xu, W., Khairallah, R., Barrows, B., . . . Stanley, W. (2008). Fish oil, but not flaxseed oil, decreases inflammation and prevents pressure overload-induced cardiac dysfunction. *Cardiovascular Research,* 319-327.

Sweeteners: The Natural Alternative to Sugar

Gregersen, S., Jeppesen, P. B., Holst, J. J., & Hermansen, K. (2004). Antihyperglycemic effects of stevioside in type 2 diabetic subjects. *Metabolism,* 53(1), 73-76.

Salminen, S., Salminen, E., & Marks, V. (1982). The effects of xylitol on the secretion of insulin and gastric inhibitory polypeptide in man and rats. *Diabetologia,* 22(6), 480-482.

Coconut Palm Sugar. Retrieved January 08, 2016, from http://www.diabetes.org/food-and-fitness/food/what-can-i-eat/making-healthy-food-choices/coconut-palm-sugar.html.

Supplements

Molfino, A., Gioia, G., Fanelli, F. R., & Muscaritoli, M. (2014). The Role for Dietary Omega-3 Fatty Acids Supplementation in Older Adults. *Nutrients,* 6(10), 4058–4072.

Schwalfenberg, G. K. (2011). A review of the critical role of vitamin D in the functioning of the immune system and the clinical implications of vitamin D deficiency. *Molecular Nutrition & Food Research,* 55(1), 96-108.

Grant, W., & Holick, M. (2005). Benefits and Requirements of Vitamin D for Optimal Health: A Review. *Alternative Medicine Review,* 10(2), 94-111.

Gill, H. S., & Guarner, F. (2004). Probiotics and human health: a clinical perspective. *Postgraduate Medical Journal,* 80(947), 516-526.

Gorbach SL. Microbiology of the Gastrointestinal Tract. In: Baron S, editor. *Medical Microbiology.* 4th edition. Galveston (TX): University of Texas Medical Branch at Galveston; 1996. Chapter 95. Available from: http://www.ncbi.nlm.nih.gov/books/NBK7670/

Labrador, M. (2013, February 25). Probiotics AND Digestive Enzymes TOGETHER. Retrieved January 6, 2016, from http://www.tacanow.org/blog/probiotics-and-digestive-enzymes-together/.

Lukaski, H. C. (2000). Magnesium, zinc, and chromium nutriture and physical activity. *The American Journal of Clinical Nutrition,* 72(2), 585s-593s.

Prasad, A. S. (2008). Zinc in human health: effect of zinc on immune cells. *Molecular Medicine,* 14(5-6), 353.

Jahnen-Dechent, W., & Ketteler, M. (2012). Magnesium basics. *Clinical Kidney Journal,* 5(Suppl 1), i3-i14.

Bucci, L., Shugarman, A., Felliciano, J., & Rodriguez, M. D. (2001). *U.S. Patent Application No.* 09/795,973.

Hoffman, J. R., Kang, J., Ratamess, N. A., Jennings, P. F., Mangine, G., & Faigenbaum, A. D. (2006). Thermogenic effect from nutritionally enriched coffee consumption. *J Int Soc Sports Nutr,* 3, 35-41.

Cannon, B., & Nedergaard, J. (2011). Nonshivering thermogenesis and its adequate measurement in metabolic studies. *The Journal of Experimental Biology,* 214(2), 242-253.

Lovallo, W. R., Whitsett, T. L., al' Absi, M., Sung, B. H., Vincent, A. S., & Wilson, M. F. (2005). Caffeine Stimulation of Cortisol Secretion Across the Waking Hours in Relation to Caffeine Intake Levels. *Psychosomatic Medicine,* 67(5), 734–739.

Mills, A. C. (2012). The effect of a BCAA supplement with and without CHO on performance in recreationally trained cyclists.

Chang C-K, Chang Chien K-M, Chang J-H, Huang M-H, Liang Y-C, Liu T-H. Branched-Chain Amino Acids and Arginine Improve Performance in Two Consecutive Days of Simulated Handball Games in Male and Female Athletes: A Randomized Trial. Tauler P, ed. *PLoS ONE.* 2015;10(3):e0121866.

Kim, L. S., Axelrod, L. J., Howard, P., Buratovich, N., & Waters, R. F. (2006). Efficacy of methylsulfonylmethane (MSM) in osteoarthritis pain of the knee: a pilot clinical trial. *Osteoarthritis and Cartilage,* 14(3), 286-294.

Grant, W., & Holick, M. (2005). Benefits and Requirements of Vitamin D for Optimal Health: A Review. *Alternative Medicine Review,* 10(2), 94-111.

The Problem of Food Intolerances and Sensitivities

Chronic Inflammation: An American Epidemic. Retrieved January 06, 2016, from http://www.mnwelldir.org/docs/terrain/chronic_inflammation.htm.

Aronson, D. (2009). Cortisol—its role in stress, inflammation, and indications for diet therapy. *Today's Dietitian,* 11(11), 38.

Hadjivassiliou, M., Grünewald, R. A., & Davies-Jones, G. A. B. (2002). Gluten sensitivity as a neurological illness. *Journal of Neurology, Neurosurgery & Psychiatry,* 72(5), 560-563.

Iablokov, V., Sydora, B. C., Foshaug, R., Meddings, J., Driedger, D., Churchill, T., & Fedorak, R. N. (2010). Naturally occurring glycoalkaloids in potatoes aggravate intestinal inflammation in two mouse models of inflammatory bowel disease. *Digestive Diseases and Sciences,* 55(11), 3078-3085.

Freed, D. L. (1999). Do dietary lectins cause disease?: The evidence is suggestive—and raises interesting possibilities for treatment. BMJ: *British Medical Journal,* 318(7190), 1023.

Cordain, L., Toohey, L., Smith, M. J., & Hickey, M. S. (2000). Modulation of immune function by dietary lectins in rheumatoid arthritis. *British Journal of Nutrition,* 83(3), 207-217.

Chait, A., & Kim, F. (2010). Saturated fatty acids and inflammation: who pays the toll? *Arteriosclerosis, Thrombosis, and Vascular Biology,* 30(4), 692-693.

Milanski, M., Degasperi, G., Coope, A., Morari, J., Denis, R., Cintra, D. E., ... & Curi, R. (2009). Saturated fatty acids produce an inflammatory response predominantly through the activation of TLR4 signaling in hypothalamus: implications for the pathogenesis of obesity. *The Journal of Neuroscience,* 29(2), 359-370.

Meet Your Metabolic Furnace

Your Digestive System and How It Works. (2013, September). Retrieved from http://www.niddk.nih.gov/health-information/health-topics/Anatomy/your-digestive-system/Pages/anatomy.aspx.

Wing, R. R., & Phelan, S. (2005). Long-term weight loss maintenance. *The American Journal of Clinical Nutrition,* 82(1), 222S-225S.

Blackburn, G. L., Phillips, J. C. C., & Morreale, S. (2001). Physician's guide to popular low-carbohydrate weight-loss diets. *Cleveland Clinic Journal of Medicine,* 68(9), 761-774.

Breaking Down Your Metabolism. Retrieved January 8, 2016, from http://www.mckinley.illinois.edu/handouts/metabolism.htm.

Exercise and aging: Can you walk away from Father Time? (2009, June 1). Retrieved January 8, 2016, from http://www.health.harvard.edu/staying-healthy/exercise_and_aging_can_you_walk_away_from_father_time.

Physical Activity and Health. (2015, June 4). Retrieved January 8, 2016, from http://www.cdc.gov/physicalactivity/basics/pa-health/.

Khan, K. M., & Scott, A. (2009). Mechanotherapy: how physical therapists' prescription of exercise promotes tissue repair. *British Journal of Sports Medicine,* 43(4), 247-252.

Carb Cycle with Sweet Potatoes: Losing the Weight, Once and for All

Fahey, T. (1998). Anabolic Steroids: Mechanisms and Effects. Retrieved January 8, 2016, from http://www.sportsci.org/encyc/anabster/anabster.html.

Insel, P., & Turner, R. (2003). *Discovering nutrition.* Sudbury, Mass.: Jones and Bartlett.

Cravings: How to Easily Defuse Them Before They Can Explode

Kravitz, L. (2008). The science of water: Nature's most important nutrient. *IDEA Fitness Journal,* 5(10), 42-49.

Jenkins, David JA, and Alexandra L. Jenkins. "Dietary fiber and the glycemic response." *Experimental Biology and Medicine* 180.3 (1985): 422-431.

The Plateau Breaker

Weight loss. (2015, January). Retrieved January 08, 2016, from http://www.mayoclinic.org/healthy-lifestyle/weight-loss/in-depth/weight-loss-plateau/art-20044615?pg=1.

Adopting the Lifestyle of Permanent Fat Loss

Shah, M., Copeland, J., Dart, L., Adams-Huet, B., James, A., & Rhea, D. (2013). Slower Eating Speed Lowers Energy Intake in Normal-Weight but not Overweight/Obese Subjects.

Foster-Powell, K., Holt, S. H., & Brand-Miller, J. C. (2002). International table of glycemic index and glycemic load values: 2002. *The American Journal of Clinical Nutrition,* 76(1), 5-56.

McCulloch, D. (2013, March 1). Dealing with Low and High Blood Sugar. Retrieved January 8, 2016, from http://www.ghc.org/healthAndWellness/?item=/common/healthAndWellness/conditions/diabetes/bloodSugar.html.

Kravitz, L. (2008). The science of water: Nature's most important nutrient. *IDEA Fitness Journal,* 5(10), 42-49.

Warburton, D. E., Nicol, C. W., & Bredin, S. S. (2006). Health benefits of physical activity: the evidence. *Canadian Medical Association Journal,* 174(6), 801-809.

Hartescu, I., Morgan, K., & Stevinson, C. D. (2015). Increased physical activity improves sleep and mood outcomes in inactive people with insomnia: a randomized controlled trial. *Journal of Sleep Research.*

Leproult, R., Copinschi, G., Buxton, O., & Van Cauter, E. (1997). Sleep loss results in an elevation of cortisol levels the next evening. Sleep: *Journal of Sleep Research & Sleep Medicine.*

Time Your Pre- and Post-Workout Nutrition with the Sweet Potato Diet

Garaulet, M., Gómez-Abellán, P., Alburquerque-Béjar, J. J., Lee, Y. C., Ordovás, J. M., & Scheer, F. A. (2013). Timing of food intake predicts weight loss effectiveness. *International Journal of Obesity* (2005), 37(4), 604.

Food as Fuel—Before, During and After Workouts. (2015). Retrieved January 8, 2016, from http://www.heart. org/HEARTORG/GettingHealthy/PhysicalActivity/FitnessBasics/Food-as-Fuel—-Before-During-and-After-Workouts_UCM_436451_Article.jsp#.VpAT-JMrJsM.

Zorzano, A., Balon, T. W., Goodman, M. N., & Ruderman, N. B. (1986). Glycogen depletion and increased insulin sensitivity and responsiveness in muscle after exercise. *American Journal of Physiology-Endocrinology and Metabolism,* 251(6), E664-E669.

Swinburn, B. A., Caterson, I., Seidell, J. C., & James, W. P. T. Diet, nutrition and the prevention of excess weight gain and obesity. *Public Health Nutrition,* 7(1A), 123-146.

Shimomura, Y., Murakami, T., Nakai, N., Nagasaki, M., & Harris, R. A. (2004). Exercise promotes BCAA catabolism: effects of BCAA supplementation on skeletal muscle during exercise. *The Journal of Nutrition,* 134(6), 1583S-1587S.

Index

kombucha, 144, 145, 272
krill oil, 145, 271–272

L

LA. *See* linoleic acid
lactobacilli, 272
lactose, 63, 77
lamb, 144
lean body mass, 12, 86
lemons, 68, 143
    juice, 144
        Lemon Garlic Sweet Potato
           Chicken, 210 (photo), 211
    in water, 40, 55
Leslie, Eliza, 15
lettuce, 143, 203, 231
Leucine, 272
limes, 40, 55, 143
    juice, 144
linoleic acid (LA), 84
lobster, 144
low fat label, 34
low-carb days, 101
    meal building for, 110
    tips for, 111–112
    training on, 265–266
Ludwig, David S., 64
lychee, 143

M

macadamia nuts, 83, 84,
    144, 241
    oil, 30, 143
macronutrients, 18, 31,
    57–58, 78, 83, 86
magnesium, 14
mahi mahi, 144
main dishes. *See* dinners
maltodextrin, 77
maltose, 77
manganese, 14

mangos, 143
maple syrup, 157, 181, 237,
    239, 243, 247
march in place exercise,
    254, 254 (photo)
Marinade, 229
Marion, Francis, 16
Mashed Ginger Sweet
    Potato, 227
Mashed Sweet Potatoes, 182
    (photo), 183, 219
Matthews, Gail, 43
mayo, 144
MCT. *See* medium chain
    triglycerides
meal portioning, 64–66
    of carbohydrates, 109
    in fat-burning cycles,
      109–111
    of fats, 109
    of flavorings, 109
    of proteins, 109
    success tips, 132
    of vegetables, 109
meals
    building, 110
    meal planner, 48–49
    meal times, 35
    preparation of, 32, 117–118
medium chain triglycerides
    (MCT), 84, 145
medium-carb days
    in carb cycling, 100–101
    fat on, 101
    meal building in, 110
    training on, 265–266
    what to eat, 100
melons, 30, 143
metabolism
    carb cycling and, 35
    metabolic effect, 94

proteins and, 78
slowing of, 8–9
weight loss and, 94
micronutrients, 57–59, 85, 86
microwaving, 141
milk
    almond, 144, 159, 239
    coconut, 161, 163, 167,
      171, 201, 239
    cow, 63–64, 87, 144
    flax seed, 144
mindset, for lasting
    success, 36
mineral water, 144
minerals, 14, 30, 57, 59, 72,
    86, 101–102
    See also specific minerals
mints, 118
moderate/leisure activities
    (aerobic) training, 264
monounsaturated fatty acids
    (MUFA), 83, 85
moods, 116
MorellisCoffee.com, 61, 273
Morning Glory plant
    family, 13
motivation, 3, 43, 45, 53, 279
mountain climbers exercise,
    258, 258 (photo)
movement
    enjoying journey, 39
    in getting started, 38–39
    success tips and, 133
mozzarella cheese, 145
MUFA. *See* monounsaturated
    fatty acids
muscle
    building, 35, 77, 93–96, 101
    carb cycling and, 34, 95
    lean tissue, 8, 81, 111, 115,
      272–273

loss, 81
preservation, 34, 272
repair of, 78
tone, 60
mushrooms, 143, 207
mussels, 144
mustard, 144
myths, 33–36

N

National Health and Nutrition
    Examination Survey, 29
natural foods, 28–29
negative stress, 44
Neural Linguistic Program-
    ming (NLP), 4
*New England Journal of
    Medicine,* 53
niacin, 14
NIH Record, 52
90/10 rule, 19, 97
NLP. *See* Neural Linguistic
    Programming
no-carb days
    in carb cycling, 101–102
    meal building in, 110
    tips for, 111–112
    training and, 265–266
    what to eat, hydration, fats
        on, 102
nutrition, 28, 52, 59
National Health and
    Nutrition Examination
    Survey, 29
on Sweet Potato Diet,
    96–97
of sweet potatoes, 14
nutrition timing
of energy-boosting
    solutions, 273–274
meaning of, 269–270

overview, 269
pre- and post-workout, 270
of protein supplements, 274
supplements in, 271–273
training and, 270–271
nuts, 34, 51, 73, 79, 132
    butters, 144, 270
    cashews, 30, 144
    peanut butter, 144, 274
    pecans, 30, 144
    pine nuts, 144
    pistachios, 144
    raw, 40, 69, 84
    roasted, 84
    as snack, 50, 69
    stocking, 52
    See also almonds; macadamia
        nuts; seeds; walnuts

O

oats, 76, 87, 145
obesity, 53
    BMI and, 25–26
    carbohydrates and, 76
    defined, 27
    as epidemic, 36
    rise of, 17
occasional foods, 40
oils
    avocado, 143
    coconut, 12, 21, 84, 143,
        155, 245
    cod liver, 145
    fish, 271–272
    flaxseed, 85
    hydrogenated, 51
    krill, 145, 271–272
    macadamia, 30, 143
    MCT, 145
    olive, 83, 85, 143, 175,
        181, 199

seed, 84
    walnut, 30, 143
Okinawan sweet potatoes,
    138
olive oil, 83, 85, 143, 175,
    181, 199
Olson, David, 3
omega-3 content, 80
The One Thing (Keller), 44
onions, 143, 201
orange sweet potatoes,
    137–138
oranges, 143, 161
oysters, 144

P

pain, 278
Paleo Diet, 2
pancakes, 158 (photo), 159
pantothenic acid, 14
papayas, 143
parsnips, 143
patience, 44–45
peaches, 143
peanut butter, 144, 274
pears, 143
peas, 80, 274
pecans, 30, 144
peppers, 13, 68, 87, 143,
    205, 213
    Enchilada Sauce, 205
    Enchiladas, 204 (photo),
        205
    Sweet Potato Chili, 168
        (photo), 169
peptides, 272
Perlmutter, David, 72
Phelps, Michael, 42
phosphorus, 14
photographic records, 45–46
pickles, 144